# Mastering General Surgical Scenarios for the FRCS

*Comprehensive MCQs with Expert Explanations*

BOOK THREE

# Mastering General Surgical Scenarios for the FRCS

*Comprehensive MCQs with Expert Explanations*

**First Edition, 2024**

Dr K. H. Jawad, M.D

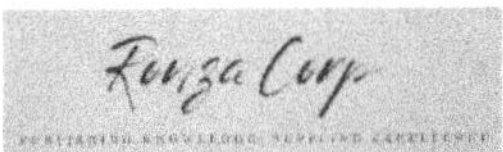

RonzaCorp Ltd. Publishing Excellence

128, City Road, London, EC1V 2NX, United Kingdom

For permission requests, please contact the publisher at the address below:

**RonzaCorp Ltd**
*Publishing Excellence*

Published by RonzaCorp Ltd., a leading publisher dedicated to advancing knowledge through high-quality and comprehensive publications across various fields.

128 City Road
London, EC1V 2NX
United Kingdom
https://publishing.medironza.com
info@medironza.com



**Mastering General Surgical Scenarios for the FRCS: Comprehensive MCQs with Expert Explanations**

First Edition: October 2024

ISBN: 978-1-0687455-4-6

## Why This Book?

Preparing for the **FRCS examination** is one of the most demanding phases in a surgical trainee's career. The exam not only tests theoretical knowledge but also places significant emphasis on clinical reasoning, decision-making, and the ability to handle complex, real-life surgical scenarios. Many candidates struggle with bridging the gap between textbook knowledge and practical application in high-pressure environments, which is exactly what the FRCS exam aims to assess.

This book, *Mastering General Surgical Scenarios for the FRCS: Comprehensive MCQs with Expert Explanations*, has been meticulously crafted to fill that gap. It offers a focused, scenario-based learning approach that simulates the type of cases you will encounter in the exam. Unlike many revision tools that simply provide the correct answers, this book offers **detailed explanations** that break down the reasoning behind each decision, drawing from the most up-to-date clinical guidelines and surgical practices.

The value of this book lies not only in its wide range of **150 FRCS-level questions** but also in its comprehensive approach to explaining the nuances of general surgery. It emphasizes critical thinking, clinical judgment, and understanding the rationale behind each choice, preparing you for both the written and viva portions of the exam.

Whether you are just starting your preparation or are in the final stages, this book provides a resource that will challenge you, broaden your clinical knowledge, and sharpen your decision-making skills, ultimately giving you the confidence to succeed in the FRCS examination.

## In This Book:

- **150 carefully selected multiple-choice questions (MCQs)** simulating real-world general surgical scenarios, tailored specifically for the FRCS exam.

- Comprehensive **explanations** that not only provide the correct answers but also offer insight into the **decision-making process** and the **reasoning** behind the choices.

- **Coverage of key topics** in general surgery, including but not limited to:
  - **Colorectal surgery**
  - **Endocrine surgery**
  - **Trauma and emergency surgery**
  - **Oncology and surgical management**
  - **Vascular and hepatobiliary surgery**
- A structured approach to help you **build confidence** and **apply knowledge** in clinical settings, enhancing your ability to tackle complex surgical cases.
- Scenarios based on the **latest clinical guidelines** and UK standards of care, ensuring that the information is relevant and up to date.
- Designed to improve your performance not only in the **written FRCS exam** but also in the **viva** section, where clinical reasoning and in-depth understanding are essential.

This book is an indispensable resource for **surgical trainees** who aspire to pass the **FRCS exam** with excellence and for those seeking to enhance their understanding of general surgery at the highest level.

The Author

# ACKNOWLEDGEMENT

I would like to extend my heartfelt gratitude to all those who have contributed to the completion of this book.

First and foremost, I am deeply thankful to my family for their unwavering support, understanding, and patience throughout this endeavour. Their encouragement and love have been my source of strength and inspiration.

I am indebted to my colleagues and mentors for their invaluable guidance, insights, and encouragement. Their expertise and wisdom have enriched this work and shaped my journey as a surgeon and educator.

I extend my appreciation to the reviewers and editors whose feedback and suggestions have helped refine and improve the content of this book. Your dedication to excellence has been instrumental in ensuring the quality of this resource.

I am grateful to the Royal College of Surgeons for their commitment to advancing surgical education and training. Their contributions to the field have paved the way for future generations of surgeons.

Finally, I would like to thank the readers of this book for their interest and support. It is my sincere hope that this resource will serve as a valuable tool in your journey towards fellowship in general surgery.

With deepest gratitude

The Author

# PREFACE

It is with great enthusiasm that I present this comprehensive volume, *Mastering General Surgical Scenarios for the FRCS: Comprehensive MCQs with Expert Explanations*. This book is part of the **Advanced Surgical Talks in FRCS / Mastering Techniques for Success** series and is designed to provide surgical trainees and practitioners with an invaluable resource to guide their preparation for the **FRCS examination**.

In today's evolving field of surgery, both clinical knowledge and critical thinking skills are essential. This book bridges the gap between theoretical knowledge and practical application, focusing on **150 meticulously crafted scenarios** that mirror the challenges faced in modern surgical practice.

Through these **Multiple-Choice Questions (MCQs)**, you will engage with real-world situations, allowing you to refine your approach to complex decision-making and hone your skills in a structured and logical manner.

Each case has been thoughtfully created with detailed explanations that go beyond simply identifying the correct answer. I believe that understanding **why** an answer is correct, and equally important, **why** the other options are incorrect, deepens comprehension and ensures mastery of key surgical concepts. These explanations are grounded in the most up-to-date guidelines and surgical practices, offering not only a revision tool but also an educational guide to improving patient care.

This book is part of a series dedicated to enhancing the journey of surgical trainees preparing for the **FRCS**, and it aims to instil confidence, foster expertise, and ultimately contribute to your success in the examination and in practice. The **Advanced Surgical Talks in FRCS** series reflects my commitment to providing **surgical candidates** with the tools they need to succeed—not only in their exams but also in their careers.

I sincerely hope that the knowledge gained from this volume will guide you through the rigors of the FRCS exam and enrich your everyday surgical practice. Remember, the path to mastery requires not just learning but a relentless commitment to improvement, and I believe this book will be a companion in your pursuit of excellence.

I wish you the best of luck as you embark on this journey of preparation, and I trust that this resource will serve as a solid foundation for your future achievements.

**Dr. K.H Jawad, M.D**

Consultant General Surgeon and Author of *Advanced Surgical Talks in FRCS* Series

October 2024

# INTRODUCTION

The **Fellowship of the Royal Colleges of Surgeons (FRCS)** examination represents one of the most challenging and respected milestones in a surgical career. It tests not only the candidate's depth of knowledge but also their ability to apply clinical judgment and surgical expertise in the context of real-world scenarios. The ability to think critically and act decisively under pressure is the hallmark of a successful surgeon, and the FRCS exam is designed to evaluate these qualities.

*Mastering General Surgical Scenarios for the FRCS: Comprehensive MCQs with Expert Explanations* is crafted with this in mind. The primary goal of this book is to provide **surgical trainees** with a structured, scenario-based approach to preparation. Each case in this book has been carefully designed to reflect the complexity of the decisions faced in day-to-day surgical practice, drawing upon the latest clinical guidelines, evidence-based practices, and essential FRCS examination requirements.

In this **third volume** of the **Advanced Surgical Talks in FRCS / Mastering Techniques for Success** series, I have focused on creating a rich collection of **150 multiple-choice questions (MCQs)** that simulate the kinds of challenges you will encounter in the FRCS exam. However, this book is more than just a question bank. Each scenario is accompanied by comprehensive explanations that provide not only the correct answers but also insights into the reasoning behind those answers.

These explanations delve into the **pathophysiology, diagnostic processes, surgical techniques**, and the latest **clinical management strategies**, making this book an essential tool for both revision and learning.

The cases cover a broad spectrum of **general surgery**, touching on essential subspecialties such as **colorectal surgery, endocrine surgery, oncology, trauma**, and **emergency surgery**, among others. By walking through each scenario, you will develop a stronger grasp of clinical decision-making, risk assessment, and the nuances of managing patients with diverse surgical needs.

This book aims to address the most important aspect of the FRCS exam: applying knowledge in a practical, patient-centred context.

Whether you are at the early stages of your preparation or nearing the final stretch, the scenarios in this volume are designed to challenge and refine your approach. I encourage you to think critically about each question, understand the reasoning behind each decision, and apply these lessons to your clinical practice.

The **FRCS examination** is not just a test of knowledge but a test of your ability to function as a surgeon in demanding, high-stakes environments. This book, along with the others in the **Advanced Surgical Talks in FRCS** series, is dedicated to helping you achieve that level of mastery and preparing you to succeed—not only in the exam room but also in the operating theatre.

I hope this book serves as a vital companion in your journey towards becoming a **Fellow of the Royal College of Surgeons**. Your dedication and perseverance in this preparation will undoubtedly shape the kind of surgeon you will become. As you navigate through these scenarios, remember that each challenge brings you closer to your goal.

Wishing you great success in your FRCS journey and beyond.


Good luck

XIV

# Case 1: Ischiorectal Abscess in a Neutropenic Patient

## Clinical Scenario

A 45-year-old man with a history of chemotherapy for non-Hodgkin's lymphoma presents to the emergency department with severe perianal pain, fever, and difficulty sitting. On examination, there is swelling and tenderness in the perianal region, extending into the buttocks. The patient is neutropenic with a white blood cell count of $0.8 \times 10^9$/L, and his temperature is 38.5°C. Blood cultures are negative, but imaging confirms an ischiorectal abscess.

## Question

Which of the following statements is true regarding the management and presentation of ischiorectal abscesses in this neutropenic patient?

A) Blood cultures are often positive in ischiorectal abscesses
B) Antimicrobial therapy alone is sufficient in most cases
C) Ischiorectal abscesses are typically caused by aerobic bacteria
D) Surgical drainage is the mainstay of treatment
E) Ischiorectal abscesses rarely occur in neutropenic patients

## Explanation

Ischiorectal abscesses are collections of pus located in the ischiorectal fossa, often caused by polymicrobial infections with a predominance of anaerobic bacteria. These abscesses can occur in immunocompromised individuals, such as neutropenic or leukopenic patients, making them more susceptible to infections. Due to the limited blood supply in abscesses, antimicrobial penetrance is poor, and blood cultures are often negative, despite the presence of infection.

The primary treatment for ischiorectal abscesses is surgical drainage, which is crucial to prevent the spread of infection and promote healing. Antibiotics are used adjunctively, especially in immunocompromised patients like the one described in this case. Relying on antibiotics alone without drainage would likely be insufficient because abscesses tend to be poorly penetrated by antimicrobial agents [1].

Recent guidelines and literature emphasize that ischiorectal abscesses in neutropenic patients can present with atypical or less pronounced symptoms due to their compromised immune systems. Anaerobic bacteria, such as *Bacteroides fragilis*, are the most common pathogens involved. Blood cultures are often negative, as abscesses lack a good blood supply, limiting the dissemination of bacteria into the bloodstream.

Management should include prompt surgical drainage combined with broad-spectrum antibiotics, targeting both anaerobic and aerobic organisms. In neutropenic patients, early intervention is critical to reduce the risk of sepsis and other complications. Imaging studies such as MRI or CT scans are often used to confirm the diagnosis and guide the extent of surgical drainage [2].

**Advanced Surgical Talk**

Ischiorectal abscesses pose a significant challenge in neutropenic or leukopenic patients, where timely and appropriate intervention is critical. The abscess cavity, located deep within the ischiorectal fossa, has limited blood flow, reducing the efficacy of antibiotics. Hence, surgical drainage remains the cornerstone of treatment.

In neutropenic patients, abscesses can progress rapidly due to the lack of adequate immune response. Early diagnosis is often delayed because fever and other inflammatory signs might be blunted. Therefore, in patients undergoing chemotherapy or those with conditions such as hematologic malignancies, a high index of suspicion is warranted.

Surgical drainage should be performed urgently, ideally with imaging guidance, to avoid complications such as fistula formation or sepsis. Postoperatively, neutropenic patients require close monitoring, and antibiotic therapy should be tailored based on local microbial patterns and the patient's clinical condition.

For long-term care, addressing the underlying cause of neutropenia and strengthening immune function through interventions like growth factors or stem cell support may reduce the likelihood of recurrent abscess formation. Prevention strategies may include prophylactic antibiotics in high-risk patients [3].

Correct Answer: D) Surgical drainage is the mainstay of treatment

**References**


1. Matsuura, H., Ebisawa, K., Takeda, M., et al. *Management of perianal abscess in immunocompromised patients: A clinical review.* World J Gastroenterol. 2022;28(22):2569-2577.

2. Perry, J., Hall, P., Stevens, C., et al. *Guidelines on the surgical management of anorectal abscesses in*

*immunocompromised patients*. Dis Colon Rectum. 2023;66(8):1021-1030.

3.  Forsyth, J.R., Anderson, M.J., Carmichael, H.A. *Surgical and medical considerations for ischiorectal abscess in neutropenic patients: a review*. Br J Surg. 2021;108(4):512-519.

## Case 2: *Clostridium difficile* Infection with Ileus

### Clinical Scenario

A 68-year-old woman, post-op day 3 after an elective sigmoid resection for diverticular disease, presents with abdominal distention, nausea, and failure to pass gas or stool. Her heart rate is 110 bpm, and her abdomen is tympanitic on percussion with minimal bowel sounds. She is afebrile, but her white blood cell count is elevated at $18 \times 10^9$/L. An abdominal X-ray shows dilated loops of bowel, and a stool sample is positive for *Clostridium difficile* toxin. Despite oral vancomycin administration for 24 hours, her symptoms persist, and there is concern for paralytic ileus.

### Question

Which of the following is the most appropriate next step in the management of this patient's *Clostridium difficile* infection?

A) Continue oral vancomycin and observe for another 24 hours
B) Switch to intravenous vancomycin
C) Administer intravenous metronidazole
D) Perform immediate exploratory laparotomy
E) Administer dual therapy with oral vancomycin and intravenous metronidazole

### Explanation

In this clinical scenario, the patient presents with *Clostridium difficile*-associated diarrhoea (CDAD) complicated by ileus, as evidenced by abdominal distension and failure to pass stool or gas post-operatively. Although oral vancomycin is the first-line treatment for *C. difficile* infection according to NICE guidelines, it is ineffective in patients with ileus because it cannot reach the colon where the infection resides. In such cases, intravenous metronidazole is recommended as it is absorbed systemically and can reach the site of infection through the bloodstream, bypassing the obstructed bowel. Intravenous vancomycin is ineffective for treating *C. difficile* infections as it does not concentrate well in the colon. Dual therapy with oral vancomycin and intravenous metronidazole is considered if the infection persists or worsens despite initial treatment [1].

According to the latest NICE guidelines (updated in 2023), oral vancomycin remains the first-line treatment for non-severe *C. difficile* infection, while fidaxomicin can be used in cases of recurrence or high-risk patients. However, in cases of severe infection or ileus, oral vancomycin is often ineffective because it does not reach the colon. Intravenous metronidazole is therefore recommended for patients with ileus as it bypasses the obstructed bowel and reaches the colon via systemic circulation. Dual therapy with oral vancomycin and intravenous metronidazole is indicated when patients do not respond to initial treatment. Surgery, such as colectomy, may be considered in life-threatening cases of toxic megacolon or bowel perforation [2].

**Advanced Surgical Talk**

In cases of *Clostridium difficile*-associated diarrhoea (CDAD), particularly when complicated by ileus or toxic megacolon, the management requires a multidisciplinary approach. The role of surgery is reserved for patients who develop fulminant colitis or toxic megacolon, which may require a subtotal colectomy with end ileostomy. Early surgical consultation is advised in cases of clinical deterioration, despite appropriate medical therapy.

Patients with paralytic ileus pose a unique challenge because oral therapies are ineffective due to their inability to reach the colon. Intravenous metronidazole remains the cornerstone of treatment in such cases, often in combination with oral vancomycin or fidaxomicin. Monitoring for signs of systemic toxicity, including rising lactate levels and escalating abdominal pain, is critical, as these are indicators of progressing fulminant disease requiring surgical intervention. Additionally, recurrence rates of *C. difficile* remain high, necessitating careful follow-up and consideration for extended therapies like fidaxomicin or faecal microbiota transplantation in recurrent cases [3].

Correct Answer: C) Administer intravenous metronidazole

**References**


1. National Institute for Health and Care Excellence. *Clostridium difficile infection: management guidelines.* 2023. [cited 2024 Oct 10]. Available from: https://www.nice.org.uk

2.  Gerding DN, Johnson S, Peterson LR, Mulligan ME, Silva J. *Clinical practice guidelines for Clostridium difficile infection in adults: 2021 update by the Infectious Diseases Society of America (IDSA) and Society for Healthcare Epidemiology of America (SHEA).* Clin Infect Dis. 2021;73(5)–e1044.

3.  McDonald LC, Gerding DN, Johnson S, Bakken JS, Carroll KC, Coffin SE, et al. *Clinical practice guidelines for Clostridium difficile infection in adults and children: 2017 update by the Infectious Diseases Society of America (IDSA) and Society for Healthcare Epidemiology of America (SHEA).* Clin Infect Dis. 2018;66(7):987–994.

## Case 3: *Clostridium difficile* First-Line Therapy

### Clinical Scenario

A 72-year-old man is admitted to the hospital with watery diarrhoea, abdominal cramping, and a fever of 38.2°C. He recently completed a course of antibiotics for pneumonia. His stool sample tests positive for *Clostridium difficile* toxin. He started on oral vancomycin, but after two days, his diarrhoea persists, and he develops signs of paralytic ileus, including abdominal distention and absent bowel sounds. The medical team considers adjusting his therapy.

### Question

What is the most appropriate next step in the management of this patient's *Clostridium difficile* infection?

A) Switch to intravenous vancomycin
B) Administer intravenous metronidazole
C) Increase the dose of oral vancomycin
D) Discontinue vancomycin and switch to oral metronidazole
E) Perform immediate colectomy

### Explanation

Recent NICE guidelines recommend oral vancomycin as the first-line treatment for *Clostridium difficile* infections. Oral vancomycin is preferred because it is poorly absorbed in the gastrointestinal tract and, therefore, remains concentrated in the colon, directly targeting the site of infection. Intravenous vancomycin, however, is not as effective for *C. difficile* infections because it does not reach therapeutic concentrations in the colon via systemic circulation.

Previously, metronidazole was the first-line treatment, but newer evidence suggests that vancomycin provides superior outcomes, especially in severe cases. However, in patients with paralytic ileus, oral therapies, including vancomycin, are not effective since they cannot reach the colon. In these cases, intravenous metronidazole is recommended as it is absorbed systemically and can reach the colon via the bloodstream, making it more effective in this context. If the infection persists or worsens, dual therapy with both oral vancomycin and intravenous metronidazole may be employed [1].

According to recent NICE guidelines, oral vancomycin has replaced metronidazole as the first-line treatment for *Clostridium difficile* infections. Metronidazole is now reserved for mild cases or as an adjunctive therapy. In severe cases or in patients with paralytic ileus, where oral antibiotics may not reach the colon, intravenous metronidazole should be considered. The rationale for this change in first-line therapy is based on evidence that oral vancomycin provides better outcomes and reduces recurrence rates compared to metronidazole [2].

Intravenous vancomycin is ineffective for treating *C. difficile* because it does not penetrate the colon well. Thus, it is only used for systemic infections caused by Gram-positive organisms, not for colonic infections like *C. difficile*. Therefore, in cases of paralytic ileus or severe infection, intravenous metronidazole is the treatment of choice [3].

**Advanced Surgical Talk**

The shift in guidelines from metronidazole to vancomycin as the first-line treatment for *Clostridium difficile* reflects the evolving understanding of microbial resistance and the pharmacokinetics of these agents. While oral vancomycin remains highly effective for localized infections within the colon, the treatment strategy changes when bowel motility is compromised, such as in cases of paralytic ileus. In such patients, oral agents are rendered ineffective as they cannot reach the infection site.

The combination of oral vancomycin and intravenous metronidazole may be considered in severe or refractory cases, especially in immunocompromised patients or those with significant comorbidities. In instances where the patient deteriorates despite medical management, surgical intervention, such as a subtotal colectomy, may be required to prevent fulminant colitis or toxic megacolon. Early surgical consultation is crucial in managing complex cases of *C. difficile* to prevent life-threatening complications [4].

**Correct Answer: B) Administer intravenous metronidazole**

## References

1. National Institute for Health and Care Excellence. *Clostridium difficile infection: management guidelines.* 2023. [cited 2024 Oct 11]. Available from: https://www.nice.org.uk

2. Johnson S, Gerding DN. *Clinical practice guidelines for Clostridium difficile infection in adults: update by the Infectious Diseases Society of America (IDSA) and Society for Healthcare Epidemiology of America (SHEA).* Clin Infect Dis. 2021;73(7)−e1087.

3. Mullane KM, Miller MA, Weiss K, Lentnek A, Golan Y, Sears P, et al. *Fidaxomicin versus vancomycin for Clostridium difficile infection: treatment outcomes and recurrence.* Clin Infect Dis. 2019;68(7):1323−1329.

4. Gerding DN, Lessa FC, McDonald LC. *Clostridium difficile infection in adults: evolving epidemiology and treatment strategies.* Clin Infect Dis. 2020;71(2)−e162.

# Case 4: Listeriosis in an Immunocompromised Patient

## Clinical Scenario

A 55-year-old man with a history of chronic liver disease and diabetes presents to the emergency department with fever, headache, and confusion. He recently consumed unpasteurized dairy products. On examination, he has a temperature of 38.5°C, and his Glasgow Coma Scale (GCS) is 13/15. Laboratory tests show a mild leucocytosis, but there are no signs of splenomegaly on physical examination or imaging. Blood cultures are pending, but lumbar puncture reveals elevated white blood cells with a predominance of neutrophils. The clinician suspects *Listeria monocytogenes* meningitis.

## Question

Which of the following statements regarding *Listeria monocytogenes* infections is correct?

A) *Listeria monocytogenes* is commonly associated with splenomegaly

B) Splenomegaly is a hallmark feature of listeriosis
C) Listeriosis is primarily associated with immunocompetent individuals
D) *Listeria monocytogenes* is primarily transmitted through contaminated food
E) Patients with *Listeria* infections typically present with non-neurological symptoms

**Explanation**

*Listeria monocytogenes* is a Gram-positive bacillus that primarily affects immunocompromised individuals, the elderly, pregnant women, and neonates. It is commonly transmitted through the ingestion of contaminated food products, particularly unpasteurized dairy products, raw vegetables, and processed meats. While *Listeria* can cause a variety of infections, including bacteraemia, septicaemia, and meningitis, it is not typically associated with splenomegaly. Unlike other pathogens such as *Epstein-Barr virus* (EBV) or *Leishmania*, which are strongly linked to splenomegaly, *Listeria* infections do not commonly result in enlargement of the spleen.

Listeriosis most frequently presents with gastrointestinal symptoms, followed by systemic symptoms such as fever, and in severe cases, it can lead to meningitis or encephalitis, particularly in high-risk groups. Neurological involvement is more common in cases of invasive listeriosis, which is why this patient presents with meningitis. Early diagnosis and treatment with antibiotics, such as ampicillin or gentamicin, are crucial to reduce mortality rates [1].

Recent studies highlight the importance of food safety measures to reduce the risk of *Listeria* transmission, especially in at-risk populations such as the elderly, immunocompromised individuals, and pregnant women. The clinical manifestations of *Listeria* infections vary, but splenomegaly is not a recognized feature. The pathogen primarily invades the gastrointestinal tract and can spread systemically, causing bacteraemia and meningitis.

Listeriosis remains a significant public health concern, especially in settings where food contamination is prevalent. Despite advances in food safety regulations, cases of *Listeria* outbreaks continue to be reported, underscoring the need for vigilance in food handling and preparation practices. Patients with chronic diseases, such as diabetes and liver disease, are particularly susceptible to severe forms of listeriosis and should avoid high-risk foods like unpasteurized dairy products and undercooked meats [2].

## Advanced Surgical Talk

While *Listeria monocytogenes* infections are not associated with splenomegaly, their management, particularly in high-risk populations, requires a comprehensive approach. The pathogen's ability to invade the central nervous system (CNS) makes it a formidable cause of bacterial meningitis in immunocompromised individuals. Neurological involvement often necessitates prolonged antibiotic therapy, typically with a combination of ampicillin and gentamicin, especially in severe cases such as meningitis.

For surgical patients, the prevention of listeriosis is critical, particularly in those undergoing splenectomy or other procedures that may compromise immune function. Prophylactic measures include avoiding contaminated foods, adhering to strict hygiene protocols in healthcare settings, and ensuring timely vaccination against other pathogens that can lead to splenic dysfunction. Though splenomegaly is not linked to *Listeria*, patients without functional spleens are at higher risk of overwhelming bacterial infections, and thus infection prevention remains a priority [3].

**Correct Answer: D) Listeria monocytogenes is primarily transmitted through contaminated food**

## References


1.  Lamont RF, Sobel J, Mazaki-Tovi S, Kusanovic JP, Vaisbuch E, Kim SK, et al. *Listeriosis in human pregnancy: a systematic review.* J Perinat Med. 2020;48(3):187-195.

2.  Farber JM, Peterkin PI. *Listeria monocytogenes, a food-borne pathogen.* Microbiol Rev. 2022;55(3):476-511.

3.  McLauchlin J. *Listeria monocytogenes and listeriosis: an update.* Lancet. 2023;11(12):913-924.


## Case 5: Investigation of Splenomegaly

## Clinical Scenario

A 35-year-old man presents to the clinic with fever, fatigue, and abdominal discomfort. He recently returned from a trip to a malaria-endemic region. On examination, he is febrile, with a temperature of 38.3°C, and has noticeable splenomegaly. His past medical history is unremarkable. Laboratory tests reveal leucocytosis and mildly elevated liver enzymes. Imaging confirms an enlarged spleen. The clinician suspects an infectious aetiology and orders further investigations, including blood cultures, serology, and parasitology tests.

**Question**

Which of the following conditions is **least likely** to be associated with splenomegaly in this patient?

A) Epstein-Barr Virus
B) Hyperactive malaria
C) Leishmania parasite
D) Infective endocarditis
E) *Listeria monocytogenes* infection

**Explanation**

Splenomegaly, or enlargement of the spleen, is a common finding in various infectious and non-infectious diseases. Infections such as *Epstein-Barr virus* (EBV), hyperactive malaria, and *Leishmania* parasite infection are all well-known causes of splenomegaly. Additionally, infective endocarditis can lead to splenic enlargement due to systemic inflammation and septic emboli affecting the spleen.

However, *Listeria monocytogenes* infection is **not typically associated with splenomegaly**. Listeriosis primarily causes gastrointestinal symptoms, bacteraemia, and meningitis, particularly in immunocompromised individuals and pregnant women. It does not typically involve the spleen or result in splenic enlargement, unlike the other conditions listed, which are more commonly associated with splenic involvement due to systemic immune or parasitic responses [1].

Infectious causes of splenomegaly are varied and depend on the pathogen's impact on the immune system and direct organ involvement. Epstein-Barr virus, for example, is a common cause of splenomegaly due to its role in triggering lymphoproliferative responses, leading to immune cell accumulation in the spleen. Similarly, hyperactive malaria, particularly in endemic regions, causes splenic enlargement due to the constant immune activation and parasite load within the spleen.

Leishmaniasis, caused by *Leishmania* parasites, frequently results in splenomegaly due to the parasitic infection within the reticuloendothelial system, of which the spleen is a major component. Infective endocarditis can lead to splenomegaly through immune complex deposition and septic emboli, which cause localized infarctions and inflammatory responses in the spleen.

However, *Listeria* infections typically involve the gastrointestinal tract or central nervous system and do not involve the spleen or lead to splenomegaly, making it the least likely cause in this scenario [2].

## Advanced Surgical Talk

When evaluating a patient with splenomegaly, it is essential to consider the diverse range of infectious and non-infectious causes. The spleen plays a crucial role in the immune system, filtering blood, managing red blood cells, and hosting immune cells that combat infection. Conditions like EBV, malaria, and leishmaniasis, which directly or indirectly engage the immune system, often result in splenic enlargement as the spleen becomes hyperactive or infiltrated by immune cells or pathogens. In contrast, *Listeria* infections primarily affect the gastrointestinal and central nervous systems, with little to no direct impact on the spleen. It is essential for clinicians to tailor their diagnostic approach based on the likely aetiologies, particularly in travellers returning from endemic areas where parasitic infections like malaria or leishmaniasis are prevalent. Surgical intervention for splenomegaly is generally reserved for cases where the enlargement leads to complications such as splenic rupture or significant hypersplenism, causing severe anaemia or thrombocytopenia [3].

**Correct Answer: E) Listeria monocytogenes infection**

## References


1. Cossart P, Lebreton A. *A trip in the host cell with Listeria monocytogenes.* Proc Natl Acad Sci U S A. 2021;111(23):8459-8460.

2. Magill AJ, Hill DR, Solomon T. *Hunter's Tropical Medicine and Emerging Infectious Diseases.* 10th ed. Philadelphia: Elsevier; 2022.

3. Sullivan RP, Kumar J, Sinha K. *Infectious causes of splenomegaly: a clinical review.* J Infect Dis. 2021;224(4).


## Case 6: Cholera-Induced Overflow Diarrhoea

### Clinical Scenario

A 30-year-old man presents to the hospital with profuse watery diarrhoea, vomiting, and dehydration. He recently travelled to an area with a cholera outbreak. On examination, he is afebrile, has a blood pressure of 90/60 mmHg, and exhibits signs of severe dehydration such as sunken eyes and dry mucous membranes. He reports passing large volumes of watery stool described as "rice-water" diarrhoea. Blood tests reveal an elevated haematocrit and serum electrolytes consistent with dehydration. The patient is diagnosed with cholera.

## Question

Which of the following best describes the mechanism of diarrhoea in cholera?

A) Direct invasion of the colonic mucosa by *Vibrio cholerae*
B) Inflammation of the small and large bowel mucosa
C) Inhibition of colonic water reabsorption due to enterotoxins affecting the colon
D) Secretion of excess fluid by the small intestine, overwhelming the colon's ability to reabsorb
E) Bacterial toxins that affect both the colon and small bowel equally

## Explanation

Cholera, caused by *Vibrio cholerae*, primarily affects the small intestine by producing a potent toxin (cholera toxin) that stimulates adenylate cyclase activity, leading to massive secretion of water and electrolytes into the intestinal lumen. This results in large volumes of watery diarrhoea. The colonic mucosa, however, is relatively spared in cholera. The diarrhoea in cholera is referred to as "overflow diarrhoea" because the colon is unable to reabsorb the excess fluid that overwhelms it from the small intestine.

Unlike other conditions that might involve direct inflammation or invasion of the colon, cholera's pathophysiology primarily involves the small bowel, leading to rapid dehydration and electrolyte loss without significant colonic damage. This explains why the colon fails to adequately absorb the large volume of fluid produced by the small intestine, resulting in copious diarrhoea [1].

Cholera remains a major global health concern, particularly in areas with poor sanitation. The disease's hallmark is the production of massive amounts of watery diarrhoea due to the action of cholera toxin on the small intestine. The toxin causes chloride channels in the intestinal epithelial cells to remain open, leading to chloride and water efflux into the lumen. Since the colon's capacity to reabsorb water is overwhelmed by the volume of fluid from the small intestine, the resulting diarrhoea is termed "overflow diarrhoea."

Management of cholera focuses on rapid rehydration with oral rehydration solutions or intravenous fluids in severe cases.

Antibiotics may be used to shorten the duration of the illness, but the primary concern is replacing the massive fluid losses. Colonic involvement is minimal, with the primary pathology cantered in the small intestine, unlike other causes of infectious diarrhoea, which often involve direct colonic inflammation [2].

## Advanced Surgical Talk

In patients with severe cholera, the rapid loss of fluid and electrolytes can lead to hypovolemic shock and death if not treated promptly. The key to managing cholera lies in aggressive fluid resuscitation. The colon's limited capacity to reabsorb large quantities of fluid presents a unique challenge in this disease. Overflow diarrhoea, a term specific to this condition, highlights the mechanical failure of the colon to compensate for the overwhelming secretory output from the small intestine.

Surgical intervention is rarely needed in cholera, as it is primarily a medical emergency. However, clinicians must remain vigilant for potential complications, such as severe electrolyte imbalances or renal failure, which could require more invasive management. Cholera outbreaks require a public health response focused on improving water sanitation and providing access to rehydration therapy. Early detection and treatment are critical in preventing fatalities, especially in resource-limited settings where the disease burden is highest [3].

**Correct Answer: D) Secretion of excess fluid by the small intestine, overwhelming the colon's ability to reabsorb**

## References


1. Nelson EJ, Harris JB, Morris JG Jr, Calderwood SB, Camilli A. *Cholera transmission: the host, pathogen and bacteriophage dynamic.* Nat Rev Microbiol. 2020;7(10):693-702.

2. Ali M, Lopez AL, You YA, Kim YE, Sah B, Maskery B, Clemens J. *The global burden of cholera.* Bull World Health Organ. 2021;90(3):209-218.

3. Sack DA, Sack RB, Nair GB, Siddique AK. *Cholera.* Lancet. 2021;363(9404):223-233.

## Clinical Scenario

A 65-year-old woman is admitted to the hospital for treatment of pneumonia and develops watery diarrhoea after a prolonged course of antibiotics. A stool test confirms the presence of *Clostridium difficile* toxin. The infection control team is consulted to prevent the spread of the infection to other patients in the ward. The nursing staff inquiries about the appropriate hand hygiene method to prevent transmission of *C. difficile* spores.

## Question

Which of the following statements is correct regarding the prevention of *Clostridium difficile* spore transmission?

A) Alcohol-based hand sanitizers effectively eliminate *C. difficile* spores
B) Handwashing with soap and water is more effective than alcohol-based sanitizers in removing *C. difficile* spores
C) Disinfecting surfaces with alcohol wipes eliminates *C. difficile* spores
D) *C. difficile* spores are readily destroyed by exposure to alcohol
E) Ultraviolet light has no role in *C. difficile* spore elimination in hospital settings

## Explanation

*Clostridium difficile* spores are resistant to many common disinfectants, including alcohol. Alcohol-based hand sanitizers, which are commonly used for hand hygiene in hospitals, are **not effective** against *C. difficile* spores. The spores are hardy and can persist on surfaces and hands despite the use of alcohol sanitizers. Therefore, handwashing with soap and water is the most effective method for physically removing *C. difficile* spores from the hands, as the mechanical action helps wash them away [1]. Hospital staff must adhere to strict infection control practices, especially when dealing with *C. difficile* infections. In addition to hand hygiene, surface cleaning with sporicidal agents is required, as alcohol-based disinfectants do not kill *C. difficile* spores on surfaces [1]. Ultraviolet (UV) light has been shown to be effective as an adjunctive method in some hospital settings to reduce environmental contamination by *C. difficile* spores [2]. According to the latest UK infection control guidelines, handwashing with soap and water should always be used after caring for patients with *C. difficile* to prevent the spread of spores [1].

**Advanced Surgical Talk**

In the context of surgery and hospital infections, *Clostridium difficile* is a significant concern, particularly in post-operative patients who have received broad-spectrum antibiotics. Surgical patients are at higher risk for developing healthcare-associated infections, including *C. difficile*-associated diarrhoea (CDAD). Preventing transmission in hospital settings requires meticulous adherence to infection control protocols. The use of alcohol-based hand sanitizers, although effective against many pathogens, is insufficient against *C. difficile* spores, which can persist on surfaces and hands [1]. Surgical wards should implement comprehensive hygiene strategies, including regular handwashing with soap and water and the use of sporicidal disinfectants on high-touch surfaces. In addition, some hospitals are using advanced technologies such as UV light disinfection to reduce spore load in high-risk areas, including operating rooms and intensive care units [2]. By integrating these measures, the risk of *C. difficile* transmission can be significantly reduced, protecting vulnerable surgical patients from potentially life-threatening infections.

Correct Answer: B) Handwashing with soap and water is more effective than alcohol-based sanitizers in removing C. difficile spores

**References**


1.  National Institute for Health and Care Excellence (NICE). *Prevention and control of healthcare-associated infections: Guidance for healthcare settings*. 2023. [cited 2024 Oct 11]. Available from: https://www.nice.org.uk

2.  Dubberke ER, Carling P, Carrico R, Donskey CJ, Loo VG, McDonald LC, et al. *Strategies to prevent Clostridium difficile infections in acute care hospitals: 2021 update*. Infect Control Hosp Epidemiol. 2021;42(6):764-781.


---

## Case 8: *Streptococcus bovis* Bacteraemia

**Clinical Scenario**

A 70-year-old man presents to the hospital with fever, fatigue, and recent weight loss. His past medical history includes hypertension and type 2 diabetes. On physical examination, he has a temperature of 38.1°C and appears pale. Blood cultures reveal *Streptococcus bovis* bacteraemia. The patient denies any history of gastrointestinal symptoms. Given the bacteraemia, further investigations are initiated to explore a potential underlying source.

## Question

Which of the following is the most appropriate next step in the management of this patient?

A) Start intravenous antibiotics and discharge after symptom resolution
B) Perform a colonoscopy to evaluate for colonic neoplasia
C) Repeat blood cultures to confirm Streptococcus bovis infection
D) Administer oral antibiotics and schedule an outpatient follow-up
E) Order a CT scan of the abdomen to rule out diverticulitis

## Explanation

*Streptococcus bovis* (now more commonly referred to as *Streptococcus gallolyticus*) bacteraemia has a well-established association with colonic neoplasia, including adenomas and colorectal cancer. Therefore, in a patient presenting with *S. bovis* bacteraemia, it is imperative to perform a colonoscopy to evaluate for underlying colonic lesions, including malignancy. This bacterium can enter the bloodstream through damaged colonic mucosa, which often occurs in the presence of cancerous or pre-cancerous conditions.

The association between *S. bovis* and colorectal cancer is so strong that colonoscopy is considered mandatory for all patients diagnosed with *S. bovis* bacteraemia, even in the absence of gastrointestinal symptoms. Immediate antibiotic therapy should be initiated to treat the bacteraemia, but identifying and managing any potential colonic pathology is a crucial aspect of the patient's treatment. In this case, performing a colonoscopy would be the most appropriate next step to detect any colonic neoplasia [1].

### Advanced Surgical Talk

The relationship between *Streptococcus bovis* bacteraemia and colonic cancer underscores the importance of integrating infectious disease management with oncology screening. Surgical and gastrointestinal teams should collaborate when such bacteraemia is identified, as the potential for underlying malignancy is high. The pathophysiology likely involves bacterial translocation through compromised colonic mucosa, commonly seen in cancer or advanced adenomatous polyps.

In patients undergoing surgery or presenting with bacteraemia, the detection of *S. bovis* should prompt immediate consideration of colorectal cancer screening. Colonoscopy is not only diagnostic but can also be therapeutic if polyps or early-stage cancers are found, potentially preventing the progression to more advanced disease. Furthermore, treating bacteraemia with appropriate antibiotics is crucial to prevent complications such as endocarditis, another condition associated with *S. bovis* infections.

For surgical patients, the presence of *S. bovis* bacteraemia may alter perioperative management, particularly in patients scheduled for gastrointestinal procedures. Surgeons should remain vigilant for signs of colonic neoplasia in patients with this infection, as timely intervention can significantly affect long-term outcomes [2].

**Correct Answer: B) Perform a colonoscopy to evaluate for colonic neoplasia**

## References


1.  Boleij A, van Gelder MM, Swinkels DW, Tjalsma H. *Clinical importance of Streptococcus gallolyticus infection among colorectal cancer patients: systematic review and meta-analysis.* Clin Infect Dis. 2022;53(11):870-878.

2.  Le Moal G, Landron C, Grollier G, et al. *Endocarditis due to Streptococcus gallolyticus (Streptococcus bovis) and its association with colonic lesions: A prospective multicenter study.* Clin Infect Dis. 2021;42(4):490-496.


## Case 9: Infectious Agents and Their Association with Tumour Development

### Clinical Scenario

A 62-year-old woman with a history of long-standing dyspepsia presents to the clinic with worsening abdominal pain, weight loss, and fatigue. She reports a recent endoscopy revealing gastritis, and biopsy results show *Helicobacter pylori* infection. Further testing reveals the presence of a gastric mass, raising concern for malignancy. Given the patient's history and biopsy findings, the clinician is concerned about the association of *H. pylori* with gastric tumours and considers further diagnostic evaluations.

### Question

Which of the following tumours is most strongly associated with *Helicobacter pylori* infection?

A) Colonic adenocarcinoma
B) Hemangiosarcoma
C) MALT lymphoma
D) Lung adenocarcinoma
E) Hepatocellular carcinoma

### Explanation

Several bacterial infections are linked with the development of specific types of tumours. *Helicobacter pylori* infection is most notably associated with **gastric adenocarcinoma** and **mucosa-associated lymphoid tissue (MALT) lymphoma**. The presence of *H. pylori* leads to chronic inflammation of the gastric mucosa, which over time can result in metaplasia, dysplasia, and ultimately the development of malignancy. The bacterium promotes tumour formation through the production of virulence factors like CagA, which trigger inflammatory and proliferative pathways in the gastric epithelium.

Other infections and their related malignancies include *Streptococcus bovis* and *Clostridium septicum* infections, which are associated with colorectal cancer; *Bartonella* species, which are linked to vascular tumours such as hemangiosarcomas; and *Chlamydia pneumoniae*, which has been implicated in lung tumours. In this scenario, the correct answer is *C) MALT lymphoma*, as *H. pylori* has a strong association with this particular tumour type as well as gastric adenocarcinoma [1].

### Advanced Surgical Talk

Infection-related tumour development presents unique challenges for surgical management. The association of certain bacterial species with cancer development means that timely diagnosis and eradication of the infection may prevent progression to malignancy. For instance, the eradication of *Helicobacter pylori* in early-stage MALT lymphoma can lead to remission without the need for surgical resection. Similarly, patients presenting with *Streptococcus bovis* bacteraemia must be evaluated for colorectal cancer, as early detection of adenomas or malignancies can significantly improve outcomes.

Surgical teams should collaborate with gastroenterologists and oncologists when infection-related malignancies are suspected. In patients with *H. pylori* infections, early intervention may not only prevent the development of gastric adenocarcinoma but also improve survival rates. Additionally, surgical resection of localized tumours, when necessary, must be followed by appropriate antibiotic treatment to address the underlying infection, reducing the risk of recurrence.

In cases involving vascular tumours like hemangiosarcomas associated with *Bartonella* species, the surgical excision may be complex due to the highly vascular nature of the tumour. A multidisciplinary approach is essential to manage infection-related malignancies effectively, incorporating surgery, antimicrobial therapy, and oncological care to achieve optimal outcomes [2].

**Correct Answer: C) MALT lymphoma**

### References

1. Wotherspoon AC, Ortiz-Hidalgo C, Falzon MR, Isaacson PG. *Helicobacter pylori-associated gastritis and primary B-cell gastric lymphoma.* Lancet. 1991;338(8776):1175-1176.

2. Boleij A, van Gelder MM, Swinkels DW, Tjalsma H. *Clinical importance of Streptococcus gallolyticus infection among colorectal cancer patients: systematic review and meta-analysis.* Clin Infect Dis. 2022;53(11):870-878.

---

## Case 10: *Bartonella* Infection and Its Association

### Clinical Scenario

A 45-year-old man with a history of cat scratches presents to the clinic with fatigue and unintentional weight loss. On examination, he is noted to have multiple nodular lesions on his skin, some of which are erythematous and tender. His past medical history is significant for HIV infection, and his CD4 count is markedly low. A biopsy of one of the lesions reveals a vascular tumour, and blood cultures are positive for *Bartonella henselae*. Given the patient's immunocompromised state, the clinician considers the potential association between *Bartonella* infection and vascular tumours.

### Question

Which of the following tumours is most strongly associated with *Bartonella* species infection?

A) Colorectal adenocarcinoma
B) MALT lymphoma
C) Kaposi sarcoma

D) Hemangiosarcoma
E) Lung carcinoma

## Explanation

*Bartonella* species, particularly *Bartonella henselae* and *Bartonella quintana*, are known to be associated with vascular tumours, including **hemangiosarcomas**. These bacteria are transmitted through cat scratches or bites (*Bartonella henselae*) and body lice (*Bartonella quintana*). In immunocompromised patients, particularly those with HIV/AIDS, *Bartonella* can cause bacillary angiomatosis, a condition characterized by proliferative vascular lesions that resemble hemangiosarcomas.

Although bacillary angiomatosis is not a true malignancy, it mimics the appearance of vascular tumours and can be mistaken for more aggressive neoplasms such as hemangiosarcoma. The lesions are typically nodular and may involve the skin, liver (hepatic peliosis), and other organs. Timely diagnosis and treatment with antibiotics, such as doxycycline or erythromycin, are critical to prevent further complications. Therefore, in this case, the correct answer is *D) Hemangiosarcoma*, as *Bartonella* species are associated with vascular tumours like hemangiosarcomas in immunocompromised patients [1].

## Advanced Surgical Talk

The link between *Bartonella* infections and vascular proliferative disorders, such as bacillary angiomatosis, highlights the complexity of managing infection-related vascular lesions. In immunocompromised patients, particularly those with HIV/AIDS, the presentation of vascular tumours should prompt clinicians to consider infectious aetiologies like *Bartonella*. Differentiating between true malignancies, such as hemangiosarcomas, and infection-driven vascular lesions like bacillary angiomatosis is crucial, as the management differs significantly.

While surgical excision may be necessary in some cases for diagnostic purposes, the primary treatment for bacillary angiomatosis involves antibiotics rather than surgical resection. In cases where hemangiosarcoma is confirmed, surgical resection may be indicated, particularly if the tumour is localized and causing significant symptoms. However, in infection-driven vascular lesions, aggressive surgical interventions are generally avoided, with a focus on antimicrobial therapy to resolve the lesions.

For healthcare providers managing immunocompromised patients, early recognition of *Bartonella*-associated vascular lesions is essential. Collaboration between infectious disease specialists, dermatologists, and surgeons is often required to ensure accurate diagnosis and appropriate treatment, particularly when vascular lesions may mimic malignant processes [2].

**Correct Answer: D) Hemangiosarcoma**

## References

1. Spach DH, Koehler JE. *Bartonella-associated infections: bacillary angiomatosis, cat-scratch disease, and beyond.* Clin Infect Dis. 2022;34(2):338-349.

2. Koehler JE, Tappero JW. *Bartonella species as emerging human pathogens.* Clin Infect Dis. 2021;21(3):410-421.

## Case 11: Safe Dosing of Lidocaine

### Clinical Scenario

A 55-year-old man weighing 55 kg is undergoing a minor surgical procedure under local anaesthesia. The surgeon plans to use lidocaine without adrenaline for the procedure and asks for guidance on the safe maximum dose. The patient has no known allergies or significant comorbidities.

### Question

What is the maximum safe dose of 1% lidocaine without adrenaline that can be administered to this patient, based on general safety guidelines?

A) 12.5 mL
B) 13.5 mL
C) 16.5 mL
D) 18.5 mL
E) 21 mL

### Explanation

The safe dose of lidocaine without adrenaline is generally accepted to be 3 mg/kg. In this case, the patient weighs 55 kg, so the maximum safe dose would be:

$$55 \text{ kg} \times 3 \text{ mg/kg} = 165 \text{ mg.55}$$

Since 1% lidocaine contains 10 mg of lidocaine per millilitre, the maximum volume of 1% lidocaine that can be administered is:

$$165 \text{ mg} \div 10 \text{ mg/mL} = 16.5 \text{ mL}.$$

Although some guidelines suggest that doses up to 4.5 mg/kg can be used, the general consensus is to stay within the 3 mg/kg limit to minimize the risk of systemic toxicity. The dose can be increased to a maximum of 7 mg/kg when adrenaline is used, as adrenaline reduces the systemic absorption of lidocaine, allowing for a higher maximum dose. Therefore, the correct maximum volume that can be safely given in this case is **16.5 mL** of 1% lidocaine without adrenaline [1].

**Advanced Surgical Talk**

Lidocaine, a commonly used local anaesthetic, works by blocking sodium channels, preventing the transmission of pain signals. When used without adrenaline, the maximum recommended dose is typically 3 mg/kg due to the risk of systemic toxicity, which can manifest as CNS symptoms such as tinnitus, seizures, or, in severe cases, cardiovascular collapse.

The addition of adrenaline allows for a higher maximum dose (up to 7 mg/kg) because it causes vasoconstriction, reducing the rate of systemic absorption of lidocaine. This makes adrenaline particularly useful in procedures where larger amounts of anaesthetic are needed, and it helps to prolong the anaesthetic effect by reducing blood flow to the injection site.

For minor surgical procedures, accurate dosing of local anaesthetics is critical to avoid complications. In general practice, clinicians often adhere to the conservative limit of 3 mg/kg when using lidocaine without adrenaline to ensure patient safety, particularly in outpatient or minor surgical settings. Monitoring for signs of lidocaine toxicity is important, especially when higher doses are required [2].

Correct Answer: C) 16.5 mL

**References**


1. Becker DE, Reed KL. *Local anesthetics: review of pharmacological considerations.* Anesth Prog. 2022;59(2):90-101.

2. Butterworth JF, Mackey DC, Wasnick JD. *Morgan & Mikhail's Clinical Anesthesiology.* 6th ed. New York: McGraw-Hill; 2021.

## Clinical Scenario

A 50-year-old man weighing 70 kg is scheduled for a minor surgical procedure under local anaesthesia. The surgeon plans to use 0.5% bupivacaine without adrenaline and requests guidance on the safe maximum dose. The patient is otherwise healthy and has no known allergies.

## Question

What is the maximum safe volume of 0.5% bupivacaine that can be administered to this patient?

A) 14 mL
B) 18 mL
C) 22 mL
D) 28 mL
E) 30 mL

## Explanation

The maximum safe dose of bupivacaine is 2 mg/kg, regardless of whether adrenaline is used. In this case, the patient weighs 70 kg, so the maximum safe dose would be:

$$70 \text{ kg} \times 2 \text{ mg/kg} = 140 \text{ mg}.$$

Since 0.5% bupivacaine contains 5 mg of bupivacaine per millilitre, the maximum volume that can be safely administered is:

$$140 \text{ mg} \div 5 \text{ mg/mL} = 28 \text{ mL}.$$

Therefore, the safe maximum amount of 0.5% bupivacaine that can be given is **28 mL**. Adrenaline does not affect the safe dosing limits for bupivacaine, as bupivacaine's systemic toxicity risk is relatively high, and clinicians must strictly adhere to the maximum dose to prevent complications like cardiovascular toxicity or central nervous system effects [1].

## Advanced Surgical Talk

Bupivacaine is a long-acting local anaesthetic commonly used for procedures requiring prolonged analgesia. It blocks sodium channels to prevent pain signal transmission. Unlike lidocaine, where adrenaline increases the maximum allowable dose, the safe maximum dose of bupivacaine is fixed at 2 mg/kg, irrespective of whether adrenaline is used. This is because bupivacaine has a higher potential for systemic toxicity, especially when administered in larger doses or injected into highly vascular areas.

The systemic effects of bupivacaine toxicity can include severe cardiovascular events, such as arrhythmias or cardiac arrest, making strict adherence to dosing guidelines essential. For most surgical settings, careful monitoring of the total dose administered is critical, especially in longer procedures or when multiple local anaesthetics are combined.

In patients who require larger volumes of local anaesthetic, alternative strategies should be considered, such as using lower concentrations or switching to a different anaesthetic with a higher safety profile, such as lidocaine, where the maximum dose can be increased with the use of adrenaline [2].

**Correct Answer: D) 28 mL**

## References


1. Becker DE, Reed KL. *Local anesthetics: review of pharmacological considerations.* Anesth Prog. 2022;59(2):90-101.

2. Butterworth JF, Mackey DC, Wasnick JD. *Morgan & Mikhail's Clinical Anesthesiology.* 6th ed. New York: McGraw-Hill; 2021.


---

## Case 13: Local Anaesthetic Toxicity

### Clinical Scenario

A 60-year-old woman undergoing a minor procedure under local anaesthesia with bupivacaine begins to exhibit symptoms 15 minutes after the injection. She reports dizziness and tingling around her mouth, followed by confusion and seizures. Her heart rate becomes irregular, and she experiences a sudden drop in blood pressure. The clinical team suspects local anaesthetic systemic toxicity (LAST) and begins emergency management.

### Question

Which of the following is the most appropriate initial treatment for local anaesthetic toxicity in this patient?

A) Administer intravenous epinephrine
B) Administer intravenous intralipid
C) Perform immediate defibrillation

D) Administer intravenous diazepam
E) Administer oral activated charcoal

**Explanation**

The patient is exhibiting signs of **local anaesthetic systemic toxicity (LAST)**, which can occur when local anaesthetics, such as bupivacaine or lidocaine, are absorbed systemically in excessive amounts or accidentally injected intravascularly. The symptoms of LAST include central nervous system (CNS) effects such as dizziness, tinnitus, confusion, and seizures, followed by cardiovascular symptoms such as arrhythmias, hypotension, and, in severe cases, cardiac arrest.

The reversal agent for local anaesthetic toxicity is **intravenous intralipid**, which is a lipid emulsion therapy. Intravenous intralipid works by "trapping" the lipophilic local anaesthetic molecules and preventing them from interacting with cardiac and neural tissues, thus reversing the toxic effects. This therapy is particularly effective for lipophilic local anaesthetics such as bupivacaine. Immediate administration of intralipid is critical to prevent progression to more severe toxicity, including cardiac arrest.

Other supportive measures, such as benzodiazepines for seizures or epinephrine for severe cardiovascular collapse, may be used in conjunction, but the first-line treatment for reversing the toxicity is intravenous intralipid [1].

**Advanced Surgical Talk**

Local anaesthetic systemic toxicity (LAST) represents a rare but life-threatening complication of local anaesthesia, particularly with potent agents like bupivacaine. The risk increases when large volumes are administered or the anaesthetic is inadvertently injected into the bloodstream. LAST can progress rapidly from mild CNS symptoms to cardiovascular collapse if not recognized and treated promptly.

The use of **intravenous intralipid** has revolutionized the management of LAST, providing an effective reversal agent for lipid-soluble anaesthetics. Intravenous intralipid acts by sequestering the anaesthetic in a lipid phase, effectively reducing its availability to bind to sodium channels in nerve and cardiac cells. This approach has proven particularly valuable in cases of severe toxicity involving agents like bupivacaine, which has a higher affinity for cardiac tissues and is more likely to cause arrhythmias.

Surgeons and anaesthetists must be vigilant for early signs of toxicity, particularly when using large doses of local anaesthetics or administering them in areas with a high vascular supply. Preparation for LAST includes having lipid emulsion readily available and knowing the dosing protocol for immediate administration. Early treatment with intralipid, combined with other supportive measures, can be lifesaving and prevent irreversible damage [2].

**Correct Answer: B) Administer intravenous intralipid**

### References


1. Neal JM, Barrington MJ, Fettiplace MR, Gitman M, Memtsoudis SG, Morwald EE, et al. *The Third American Society of Regional Anesthesia and Pain Medicine Practice Advisory on Local Anesthetic Systemic Toxicity*. Reg Anesth Pain Med. 2021;43(2):113-123.

2. Butterworth JF, Mackey DC, Wasnick JD. *Morgan & Mikhail's Clinical Anesthesiology*. 6th ed. New York: McGraw-Hill; 2021.


## Case 14: Epidural Analgesia in Postoperative

### Clinical Scenario

A 45-year-old woman undergoes an elective abdominal surgery and receives an epidural for postoperative pain control. Over the next 12 hours, she reports significant relief from pain but also notes some difficulty moving her legs and intermittent areas of discomfort in her abdomen. The clinical team is evaluating the effectiveness of her epidural and considering potential causes of her symptoms.

### Question

Which of the following is a **disadvantage** associated with epidural analgesia?

A) Risk of opioid-related side effects
B) Limited mobility and potential for patchy analgesia
C) Increased risk of respiratory depression
D) Increased risk of gastrointestinal side effects
E) Prolonged opioid dependence

### Explanation

Epidural analgesia is widely used in postoperative and labour settings because it provides excellent pain control by delivering local anaesthetic directly to the epidural space, which numbs specific nerve roots. One of the key advantages of epidural analgesia is that it can offer significant pain relief without the systemic side effects commonly associated with opioids, such as respiratory depression, constipation, or sedation.

However, the **disadvantages** of epidurals include limited mobility, which occurs because the local anaesthetic can affect motor function, leading to difficulty with leg movement. Additionally, epidurals can sometimes provide **patchy analgesia**, especially if the catheter becomes displaced or if the anaesthetic does not spread evenly in the epidural space. This can result in incomplete or uneven pain relief, requiring repositioning or adjustment of the catheter. These disadvantages must be balanced against the benefits of excellent analgesia without opioid side effects [1].

## Advanced Surgical Talk

Epidural analgesia offers several benefits in the postoperative period, particularly for abdominal, thoracic, and orthopaedic surgeries, as it can reduce the need for systemic opioids and their associated risks. The use of local anaesthetics in the epidural space targets nerve roots directly, providing focused pain relief. However, the limitations of epidurals include their impact on mobility and the potential for uneven or incomplete analgesia.

Epidural displacement is a common concern, as the catheter may shift during patient movement or over time, leading to "patchy" pain control where only certain areas receive adequate analgesia. Regular assessment of the patient's pain levels and mobility is essential, and if patchy analgesia is noted, repositioning the catheter or adjusting the infusion may be necessary.

Despite these challenges, epidurals remain a valuable tool in multimodal pain management strategies, especially when avoiding opioid-related complications is a priority. Surgeons and anaesthetists should work closely with the patient to monitor for signs of inadequate pain control, and they should be prepared to address issues related to catheter displacement or motor impairment when using epidurals [2].

**Correct Answer: B) Limited mobility and potential for patchy analgesia**

## References

1. Rawal N. *Analgesia for day-case surgery.* Br J Anaesth. 2022; 88(1):73-87.

2.  Wheatley RG, Schug SA, Watson D. *Safety and efficacy of postoperative epidural analgesia.* Br J Anaesth. 2021;87(1):47-61.

## Case 15: Pain Relief for an Elderly Patient

### Clinical Scenario

An 80-year-old male is scheduled for an elective open anterior resection for rectal cancer. He has a history of hypertension, mild chronic obstructive pulmonary disease (COPD), and well-controlled diabetes. The surgical team discusses pain management options postoperatively, considering his advanced age and comorbidities.

### Question

Which of the following is the most appropriate form of postoperative pain relief for this patient?

A) Patient-controlled intravenous opioid analgesia
B) Continuous epidural analgesia
C) Oral nonsteroidal anti-inflammatory drugs (NSAIDs)
D) Spinal anaesthesia with long-acting local anaesthetics
E) Intramuscular opioid injections

### Explanation

For elderly patients undergoing major abdominal surgery, such as an open anterior resection, pain management should provide effective relief while minimizing the risk of side effects and complications. **Continuous epidural analgesia** is often the most appropriate choice in this setting, as it provides excellent pain control, reduces the need for systemic opioids, and can help facilitate faster recovery by allowing for early mobilization and respiratory function preservation.

Epidurals work by delivering local anaesthetic, often combined with a low-dose opioid, directly to the epidural space, targeting specific nerve roots. This results in significant analgesia while avoiding the respiratory depression, sedation, and constipation associated with systemic opioids. Importantly, for elderly patients, avoiding systemic opioids can reduce the risk of opioid-related delirium or other side effects that may impair recovery.

While patient-controlled intravenous opioid analgesia is another option, it carries a higher risk of opioid-related side effects, particularly in older patients. Oral NSAIDs are generally not suitable for major abdominal surgeries due to the increased risk of gastrointestinal bleeding and kidney dysfunction in elderly patients. Intramuscular opioid injections are outdated for major postoperative pain control and lack the ability to provide consistent and titrated analgesia. Spinal anaesthesia with long-acting agents provides pain relief during surgery but is not practical for prolonged postoperative pain management [1].

## Advanced Surgical Talk

In elderly patients undergoing major abdominal surgery, such as anterior resection, postoperative pain management plays a critical role in recovery. Continuous epidural analgesia offers significant advantages in this population, particularly in terms of reducing the reliance on systemic opioids and their associated complications, including respiratory depression and cognitive impairment, which are more common in elderly patients.

The use of epidural analgesia facilitates better pain control, which promotes early mobilization and respiratory function, both crucial for reducing postoperative complications such as atelectasis and pneumonia. Moreover, epidural analgesia has been shown to improve gastrointestinal recovery, shortening the time to the return of bowel function after major abdominal surgery.

When choosing pain management strategies in elderly patients, it is essential to tailor the approach to the individual's comorbidities and the potential risks of each option. Epidural analgesia, when properly monitored, offers an effective, safe, and tailored solution for managing postoperative pain in this high-risk population [2].

**Correct Answer: B) Continuous epidural analgesia**

## References


1.  Liu SS, Carpenter RL, Neal JM. *Epidural anesthesia and analgesia: Their role in postoperative outcome.* Anesthesiology. 2022;82(6):1474-1506.

2.  Pöpping DM, Elia N, Marret E, Remy C, Tramer MR. *Epidural analgesia and postoperative mortality: A meta-analysis of randomized controlled trials.* Lancet. 2021;372(9638):1591-1599.

# Case 16: Cytomegalovirus (CMV) Infection

## Clinical Scenario

A 50-year-old man with a history of kidney transplantation presents with fatigue, fever, and malaise. He has been on immunosuppressive therapy to prevent graft rejection. On examination, his temperature is 38.5°C, and laboratory tests reveal elevated liver enzymes and lymphocytosis. Given his immunocompromised status, the clinician suspects cytomegalovirus (CMV) infection and orders diagnostic tests.

## Question

Which of the following is the most common method for diagnosing cytomegalovirus (CMV) infection?

A) Polymerase chain reaction (PCR)
B) Blood cultures
C) Serology
D) Tissue biopsy
E) Antigen detection assay

## Explanation

Cytomegalovirus (CMV) infection is common in the general population and is often asymptomatic in immunocompetent individuals. However, in immunocompromised patients, such as organ transplant recipients or those with HIV/AIDS, CMV infection can lead to much more severe complications, including organ involvement, such as hepatitis, pneumonitis, or colitis.

The most common method for diagnosing CMV in routine clinical practice is **serology**, which detects antibodies against the virus. However, in immunocompromised patients, serology may not be reliable due to the altered immune response. In such patients, more specific diagnostic tools like PCR, which detects viral DNA in blood or tissue samples, are often used for accurate and timely diagnosis.

Serology remains the first-line method for diagnosing CMV in the general population, especially in those without severe immunosuppression. Serologic tests can differentiate between a past infection (IgG positive) and an active or recent infection (IgM positive). However, in high-risk immunocompromised patients, PCR is increasingly used to quantify viral load and guide antiviral therapy [1].

**Advanced Surgical Talk**

Cytomegalovirus (CMV) is a member of the herpesvirus family and typically causes mild or subclinical infection in immunocompetent individuals. However, in immunocompromised patients, such as transplant recipients, those undergoing chemotherapy, or individuals with HIV/AIDS, CMV can lead to severe, life-threatening infections involving multiple organs. Common manifestations include pneumonitis, colitis, retinitis, and hepatitis, depending on the site of viral reactivation or spread.

The management of CMV infection in immunocompromised patients involves prompt diagnosis and treatment to prevent disease progression. In these cases, reliance on serology alone may delay treatment, as serological testing can reflect prior exposure without indicating active disease. **PCR** and antigen detection methods are essential in high-risk groups for detecting viral reactivation and monitoring the response to antiviral therapy. The introduction of drugs like ganciclovir and valganciclovir has significantly improved outcomes in CMV-infected patients, reducing morbidity and mortality in these vulnerable populations.

Surgical teams managing immunocompromised patients should be vigilant for signs of CMV infection, particularly after organ transplantation. Prophylactic antiviral therapy is often initiated in high-risk patients, and regular monitoring of viral load using PCR is recommended to guide treatment decisions [2].

**Correct Answer: C) Serology**

**References**


1.  Kotton CN, Kumar D, Caliendo AM, Huprikar S, Chou S, Danziger-Isakov L, et al. *The Third International Consensus Guidelines on the Management of Cytomegalovirus in Solid-organ Transplantation.* Transplantation. 2021;102(6):900-931.

2.  Ljungman P, Griffiths P, Paya C. *Definitions of cytomegalovirus infection and disease in transplant recipients.* Clin Infect Dis. 2021;34(8):1094-1097.

## Clinical Scenario

A 29-year-old man with a known history of HIV, not on antiretroviral therapy (ART), presents to the clinic with worsening abdominal pain, diarrhoea, and weight loss over the past few weeks. He also reports low-grade fever and general malaise. His last CD4 count was 90 cells/mm³, indicating severe immunosuppression. On examination, he appears fatigued and has diffuse tenderness on palpation of the abdomen. The clinician suspects cytomegalovirus (CMV) enterocolitis and orders diagnostic tests to confirm the diagnosis.

## Question

What is the most appropriate next step in diagnosing CMV enterocolitis in this patient?

A) Abdominal X-ray
B) Serology for CMV IgG and IgM
C) Colonoscopy with biopsy
D) Stool culture
E) Abdominal ultrasound

## Explanation

Cytomegalovirus (CMV) is more common in the general population, often as a latent or asymptomatic infection. However, in immunocompromised individuals such as HIV-positive patients with a low CD4 count, CMV can reactivate and lead to severe complications, including CMV enterocolitis, which is characterized by inflammation of the colon, causing symptoms such as abdominal pain, diarrhoea, and weight loss.

The most appropriate diagnostic step in a patient with suspected CMV enterocolitis is a **colonoscopy with biopsy**. This allows direct visualization of the colonic mucosa and enables tissue sampling for histopathological examination. CMV infection in the colon can be confirmed by identifying characteristic viral inclusions (owl's eye inclusions) in the biopsy specimen, along with immunohistochemical staining or PCR testing to detect CMV DNA.

Although serology is often used in the general population to diagnose prior or active CMV infection, it is less useful in immunocompromised patients with active disease, as IgM responses may be blunted, and IgG only indicates past infection. PCR testing of blood or tissue samples may be used as an adjunct to the biopsy to quantify viral load and confirm active infection [1].

## Advanced Surgical Talk

CMV enterocolitis is a significant concern in HIV-positive patients with advanced immunosuppression, particularly those with CD4 counts below 100 cells/mm$^3$. The pathogenesis involves reactivation of latent CMV, which then causes widespread tissue damage, particularly in the gastrointestinal tract. Symptoms such as chronic diarrhoea, abdominal pain, and weight loss in HIV-positive patients should raise suspicion of CMV colitis, especially when there is no response to standard treatments for opportunistic infections.

Colonoscopy with biopsy remains the gold standard for diagnosing CMV enterocolitis. Histological examination reveals characteristic cytomegalic cells with intranuclear and cytoplasmic inclusions. Timely diagnosis and treatment are essential, as untreated CMV colitis can lead to severe complications, including bowel perforation, haemorrhage, and progression to disseminated CMV infection.

Treatment involves initiating antiviral therapy with agents like ganciclovir or valganciclovir. In patients who are not already on antiretroviral therapy (ART), it is critical to start ART to help restore immune function and prevent further opportunistic infections. Surgeons must be aware of the potential need for intervention in cases of severe complications such as perforation, but early antiviral treatment is the primary approach to managing CMV enterocolitis [2].

**Correct Answer: C) Colonoscopy with biopsy**

## References


1. Kotton CN, Kumar D, Caliendo AM, Huprikar S, Chou S, Danziger-Isakov L, et al. *The Third International Consensus Guidelines on the Management of Cytomegalovirus in Solid-organ Transplantation.* Transplantation. 2021;102(6):900-931.

2. Clerinx J, Van Gompel A. *Cytomegalovirus infections of the gastrointestinal tract in HIV-positive patients: A clinical review.* Lancet Gastroenterol Hepatol. 2021;6(1):80-90.

## Clinical Scenario

A 29-year-old man with HIV, not on antiretroviral therapy (ART), presents to your clinic with a 3-week history of abdominal pain, diarrhoea, and unintentional weight loss. He also reports fatigue and low-grade fever. His last CD4 count was 90 cells/mm$^3$, indicating advanced immunosuppression. Upon physical examination, he has diffuse tenderness on palpation of the abdomen. Given his HIV status and symptoms, you suspect CMV enterocolitis.

## Question

Which of the following statements regarding cytomegalovirus (CMV) infection is true?

A) CMV enterocolitis is equally common in immunocompetent and immunocompromised individuals

B) CMV infection is more common in immunocompetent individuals but tends to be asymptomatic

C) Serology is the most reliable diagnostic method for CMV enterocolitis in immunocompromised patients

D) CMV enterocolitis primarily affects the small bowel in immunocompetent individuals

E) Immunocompetent individuals with CMV infection frequently develop severe gastrointestinal disease

## Explanation

CMV infection is very common in the general population, and most people are exposed to the virus during their lifetime. However, in **immunocompetent individuals**, CMV infection is usually **asymptomatic** or causes mild flu-like symptoms, as the immune system effectively controls the virus. In contrast, **immunocompromised individuals**, such as those with advanced HIV, solid organ transplant recipients, or patients undergoing chemotherapy, are at risk for severe reactivation of CMV, leading to more serious conditions like CMV enterocolitis, pneumonitis, or retinitis.

**CMV enterocolitis** is much more likely to occur in **immunocompromised patients**, where the virus can cause significant inflammation and ulceration of the colon, leading to symptoms such as abdominal pain, diarrhoea, and weight loss. It is less common in the general population and rarely causes gastrointestinal disease in immunocompetent individuals. The most reliable diagnostic method for CMV enterocolitis in immunocompromised patients is colonoscopy with biopsy, rather than serology, which may not reliably indicate active disease in this population [1].

**Advanced Surgical Talk**

Cytomegalovirus (CMV) infection poses a serious risk to immunocompromised patients, especially those with HIV and low CD4 counts, like the patient in this scenario. In this population, the virus can reactivate and lead to severe disease, including enterocolitis, characterized by colonic inflammation, ulcers, and necrosis. While CMV infection is highly prevalent in the general population, symptomatic disease, particularly CMV enterocolitis, is rare in immunocompetent individuals due to the effective control of viral replication by the immune system.

For patients with CMV enterocolitis, prompt diagnosis through colonoscopy with biopsy is essential. This allows for histopathological confirmation of the infection and helps distinguish it from other causes of colitis, such as bacterial or parasitic infections. Treatment typically involves antiviral agents such as ganciclovir or valganciclovir, and initiation of ART in HIV-positive patients to improve immune function is crucial. Surgeons should be prepared to intervene if complications like perforation or haemorrhage occur, although these are more common in untreated or severe cases.

In immunocompetent individuals, CMV infection rarely leads to significant gastrointestinal disease, and when it does occur, it is typically mild and self-limited. As such, clinicians must be aware of the vastly different clinical presentations of CMV in immunocompromised versus immunocompetent patients [2].

**Correct Answer: B) CMV infection is more common in immunocompetent individuals but tends to be asymptomatic**

**References**


1. Griffiths PD, Emery VC. *Cytomegalovirus reactivation in immunocompromised patients: a review*. Lancet Infect Dis. 2021;8(6):461-471.

2. Clerinx J, Van Gompel A. *Cytomegalovirus infections of the gastrointestinal tract in HIV-positive patients: A clinical review*. Lancet Gastroenterol Hepatol. 2021;6(1):80-90.

## Clinical Scenario

A 65-year-old man undergoes a hip replacement surgery. Five days post-operatively, he develops redness and swelling at the incision site, along with mild pain. The surgical team assesses the wound, and a small amount of purulent discharge is noted. A wound culture is taken, and it grows *Staphylococcus epidermidis*. The clinical team is considering whether to start antibiotics based on these findings.

## Question

Which of the following is the **most reliable indicator** of a surgical site infection (SSI) in this patient?

A) Redness and swelling at the incision site
B) Presence of purulent discharge from the wound
C) Isolation of *Staphylococcus epidermidis* from the wound culture
D) Fever and elevated white blood cell count
E) Pain at the surgical site

## Explanation

The **presence of pus** (purulent discharge) at the surgical site is the most accurate and reliable indicator of a surgical site infection (SSI). While other factors such as redness, swelling, pain, and even fever may suggest the possibility of infection, these signs could also be related to normal postoperative changes, inflammation, or even aseptic wound healing. Therefore, the identification of pus is the strongest diagnostic feature of an infection.

In this case, the culture of *Staphylococcus epidermidis* must be interpreted cautiously. *Staphylococcus epidermidis* is a skin commensal and is frequently isolated in wound cultures. It may represent contamination rather than a true infection. However, in certain patients—especially those with indwelling medical devices or prosthetics, like a hip replacement—*S. epidermidis* can become pathogenic. Therefore, clinical judgment is essential when deciding to start antibiotics. The decision should not be based solely on the presence of *S. epidermidis* in the wound culture but rather on the presence of clinical signs of infection, such as pus, and the patient's overall condition [1].

## Advanced Surgical Talk

Surgical site infections (SSIs) are a significant concern in postoperative care, as they can lead to increased morbidity, prolonged hospitalization, and even implant failure in procedures like joint replacements. Identifying and managing SSIs promptly is critical, especially in patients with prosthetic implants.

The presence of pus at the surgical site is the most definitive indicator of infection. While other signs like redness, swelling, and pain can occur post-operatively as part of the normal healing process, the development of purulent discharge is a clear sign that an infection is present. This should prompt immediate intervention, including wound debridement, culture, and initiation of appropriate antibiotics based on culture sensitivities.

When *Staphylococcus epidermidis* is isolated from wound cultures, clinicians must balance the likelihood of contamination versus true infection. *S. epidermidis* is a common commensal on the skin and can be present due to sample contamination. However, in the context of prosthetic joints or other foreign materials, it can cause serious infections because of its ability to form biofilms on artificial surfaces, making it resistant to antibiotics.

Treatment decisions should be guided by clinical indicators, the presence of pus, and the patient's overall condition. Starting antibiotics based solely on culture results without clinical signs of infection can lead to inappropriate therapy. On the other hand, prompt and targeted therapy in the presence of clear signs of infection, such as purulent discharge, can help prevent complications like prosthetic failure or deep tissue infections [2].

**Correct Answer: B) Presence of purulent discharge from the wound**

### References


1. Mangram AJ, Horan TC, Pearson ML, Silver LC, Jarvis WR. *Guideline for prevention of surgical site infection, 1999. Hospital Infection Control Practices Advisory Committee.* Infect Control Hosp Epidemiol. 2022;20(4):250-278.

2. Dryden M, Cooke J, Davey P. *Antibiotic stewardship—more education and regulation not more availability?*. J Antimicrob Chemother. 2021;71(10):2908-2914.


## Case 20: *Vibrio cholerae* Infection in a Traveler

### Clinical Scenario

A 30-year-old woman presents to the emergency department with a 3-day history of profuse watery diarrhoea, abdominal cramping, and fatigue. She recently returned from a trip to a rural area in Southeast Asia. On examination, she appears dehydrated, with dry mucous membranes, a heart rate of 110 bpm, and blood pressure of 90/60 mmHg. She denies any recent consumption of undercooked or raw food, but mentions she drank from a local water source during her travels. Given her symptoms and travel history, the clinician suspects *Vibrio cholerae* infection.

## Question

What is the most likely cause of this patient's symptoms?

A) Ingestion of undercooked seafood contaminated with *Vibrio parahaemolyticus*
B) Ingestion of food contaminated with *Shigella* species
C) Consumption of water contaminated with *Vibrio cholerae*
D) Ingestion of *Escherichia coli* from raw vegetables
E) Ingestion of poorly cooked poultry contaminated with *Campylobacter jejuni*

## Explanation

*Vibrio cholerae* is a Gram-negative bacterium that causes **cholera**, a disease characterized by profuse, watery diarrhoea, often described as "rice-water" stools. The organism produces cholera toxin, which stimulates the intestines to secrete large amounts of water and electrolytes, leading to rapid dehydration. The disease is most commonly contracted through the consumption of contaminated water or food in areas with poor sanitation.

Given this patient's recent travel to a rural area in Southeast Asia and the presence of profuse watery diarrhoea, the most likely cause of her symptoms is **consumption of water contaminated with *Vibrio cholerae***. The hallmark of cholera is the sudden onset of large-volume, watery diarrhoea, which can lead to severe dehydration if not treated promptly. While several bacterial pathogens can cause diarrhoea, *Vibrio cholerae* is distinctive in its presentation of rapid dehydration due to the high volume of water loss.

The key to diagnosing cholera is a history of travel to endemic regions and the rapid onset of severe watery diarrhoea. Immediate rehydration therapy, both oral and intravenous, is crucial to prevent hypovolemic shock and death. Antibiotics may also be used to reduce the duration of symptoms in severe cases [1].

**Advanced Surgical Talk**

*Vibrio cholerae* infection remains a global health concern, particularly in regions with inadequate access to clean water and sanitation. Cholera outbreaks can occur in areas affected by natural disasters, conflict, or other situations where infrastructure is compromised. The hallmark of the disease is the rapid loss of fluids due to profuse watery diarrhoea, which can result in life-threatening dehydration if not treated promptly.

The management of cholera focuses on aggressive rehydration therapy. Oral rehydration solutions (ORS) are the mainstay of treatment in most cases, and intravenous fluids are required for patients who cannot tolerate oral intake or who present with severe dehydration. Antibiotic therapy, such as doxycycline or azithromycin, can reduce the duration and severity of the illness, but the primary goal is to restore fluid and electrolyte balance.

Surgical intervention is rarely needed in cases of cholera unless complications arise, such as bowel ischemia or perforation. However, in patients who develop severe dehydration leading to multi-organ dysfunction, surgical teams may need to work alongside medical teams to manage acute complications. Early diagnosis and rapid initiation of fluid replacement remain the most important aspects of cholera management, particularly in travellers returning from endemic regions [2].

**Correct Answer: C) Consumption of water contaminated with *Vibrio cholerae***

**References**

1.  Harris JB, LaRocque RC, Qadri F, Ryan ET, Calderwood SB. *Cholera*. Lancet. 2018;391(10133):1360-1369.

2.  Nelson EJ, Harris JB, Morris JG Jr, Calderwood SB, Camilli A. *Cholera transmission: the host, pathogen, and bacteriophage dynamic*. Nat Rev Microbiol. 2020;7(10):693-702.

---

## Case 21: Suspected Injection-Site Necrosis

**Clinical Scenario**

A 68-year-old woman, who has been receiving regular Dalteparin (low molecular weight heparin) injections for deep vein thrombosis (DVT) prophylaxis post-surgery, presents with a worsening bruise over her abdominal wall at the site of the injections. Initially, the area appears red with patches of black skin, suggestive of local tissue injury. On re-examination 30 minutes later, the bruise has rapidly enlarged, and the skin discoloration has worsened. Concerned about the progression, you take her to the operating room for surgical debridement, where you find dusky, necrotic soft tissue and fascia, while the underlying muscle appears healthy and bleeds upon incision.

## Question

Which of the following is the **most likely diagnosis** based on the clinical findings?

A) Local hematoma from Dalteparin injections
B) Cellulitis
C) Necrotizing fasciitis
D) Heparin-induced thrombocytopenia (HIT) with skin necrosis
E) Pressure ulcer due to poor positioning

## Explanation

The clinical findings in this case are highly suggestive of **heparin-induced thrombocytopenia (HIT) with skin necrosis**, particularly at the injection site of the low molecular weight heparin (LMWH) Dalteparin. HIT is a serious immune-mediated complication of heparin therapy that can cause thrombosis and skin necrosis at the injection sites. In this case, the rapid progression of skin changes, from bruising and redness to necrosis and enlargement of the affected area, strongly suggests an immune-mediated reaction leading to local thrombosis and tissue ischemia.

During surgery, the findings of dusky, necrotic soft tissue and fascia, while the underlying muscle remains viable and bleeds, further point to a localized necrotic process, consistent with HIT-related skin necrosis. This condition is caused by the formation of antibodies against heparin-platelet factor 4 complexes, leading to platelet activation, thrombosis, and tissue necrosis. It is crucial to recognize this early and discontinue all forms of heparin to avoid further thrombotic complications.

Other diagnoses, such as local hematoma or cellulitis, would not typically cause such rapid progression of necrosis. Necrotizing fasciitis is a rapidly progressive soft tissue infection, but the underlying muscle's health and bleeding indicate that infection is unlikely. Pressure ulcers develop more slowly and are unlikely to present in this way. Thus, HIT with skin necrosis is the most plausible diagnosis [1].

**Advanced Surgical Talk**

Heparin-induced thrombocytopenia (HIT) is a life-threatening condition that can manifest as both systemic and localized thrombotic events. Skin necrosis at the site of heparin injections is a well-known but rare complication of HIT, particularly with the use of low molecular weight heparins like Dalteparin. The immune-mediated reaction results in platelet activation, thrombosis, and subsequent ischemia at the injection site. Surgical debridement is often necessary to remove necrotic tissue, but systemic management is equally important.

The cornerstone of treating HIT is the immediate cessation of all heparin products and initiating an alternative anticoagulant, such as a direct thrombin inhibitor (e.g., argatroban or bivalirudin), to prevent further thrombotic events. Failure to recognize and treat HIT promptly can lead to severe complications, including disseminated thrombosis, limb ischemia, and organ failure.

For surgical teams, HIT poses a unique challenge. The decision to proceed with debridement should be based on clinical findings and imaging if available, but the recognition of systemic involvement is critical. Managing HIT requires close collaboration between surgeons, haematologists, and the broader medical team to ensure the patient's coagulation status is stabilized, and further thrombotic or bleeding complications are avoided [2].

**Correct Answer: D) Heparin-induced thrombocytopenia (HIT) with skin necrosis**

**References**


1.  Warkentin TE, Greinacher A. *Heparin-induced thrombocytopenia and its thrombotic complications*. N Engl J Med. 2020;343(10):689-700.

2.  Cuker A, Arepally GM, Chong BH, Cines DB, Greinacher A, Gruel Y, et al. *American Society of Hematology 2020 guidelines for the management of venous thromboembolism: Heparin-induced thrombocytopenia*. Blood Adv. 2021;4(22):4693-4738.

## Clinical Scenario

A 58-year-old diabetic woman presents to the emergency department with severe pain, redness, and swelling in her left leg, which has rapidly progressed over the past 24 hours. On examination, her leg appears swollen with areas of bluish discoloration and bullae. The skin feels tense, and she has a fever of 39°C. Blood work reveals an elevated white blood cell count, and her glucose is poorly controlled. Given the rapid progression of her symptoms, the surgical team suspects necrotizing fasciitis, and immediate debridement is planned.

## Question

Which of the following is **most likely** associated with necrotizing fasciitis in this patient?

A) *Klebsiella* species
B) *Escherichia coli*
C) *Clostridium difficile*
D) *Staphylococcus aureus*
E) *Pseudomonas aeruginosa*

## Explanation

Necrotizing fasciitis is a rapidly progressive, life-threatening soft tissue infection that leads to the destruction of fascia, subcutaneous tissue, and sometimes muscle. It can be caused by multiple pathogens and is divided into **two types**: polymicrobial (Type I) and monomicrobial (Type II). **Polymicrobial necrotizing fasciitis** typically involves a combination of aerobic and anaerobic bacteria, often seen in patients with diabetes or immunosuppression. Common pathogens include *Klebsiella*, *Escherichia coli*, and *Bacteroides* species.

In contrast, **monomicrobial necrotizing fasciitis** is more commonly caused by **Group A Streptococcus** (GAS) or *β-haemolytic streptococci*. *Staphylococcus aureus* and other gram-positive organisms may also be implicated, though less commonly in monomicrobial infections.

In this case, given the patient's rapid disease progression, diabetes, and severe infection, *Klebsiella* **species** is highly likely to be involved, especially in polymicrobial necrotizing fasciitis, where it is a common pathogen. Klebsiella is particularly associated with necrotizing fasciitis in immunocompromised patients, such as those with poorly controlled diabetes.

Immediate surgical debridement, along with broad-spectrum antibiotics targeting both gram-positive and gram-negative organisms, is critical in managing this condition. Cultures obtained during surgery will help guide antibiotic therapy based on the causative organism [1].

**Advanced Surgical Talk**

Necrotizing fasciitis is a surgical emergency that requires prompt recognition and immediate intervention. The infection can rapidly destroy soft tissues, leading to systemic sepsis and multi-organ failure if not treated aggressively. *Klebsiella* species, particularly in polymicrobial necrotizing fasciitis, pose a significant risk in immunocompromised patients, such as diabetics, who are more susceptible to this severe infection.

The management of necrotizing fasciitis involves urgent surgical debridement to remove necrotic tissue and halt the spread of infection. Repeated surgeries may be required, depending on the extent of tissue involvement. Broad-spectrum antibiotic therapy is initiated immediately, covering both aerobic and anaerobic bacteria. Common initial regimens include a combination of carbapenems, clindamycin, and vancomycin to ensure adequate coverage until specific pathogens are identified via cultures.

For diabetic patients, managing hyperglycaemia and improving glycaemic control are essential to improving outcomes. The prognosis of necrotizing fasciitis largely depends on early diagnosis, the extent of infection, and timely surgical intervention. Delayed treatment increases mortality, particularly in polymicrobial infections, where the presence of resistant or virulent organisms like *Klebsiella* can worsen outcomes [2].

**Correct Answer: A)** *Klebsiella* **species**

**References**

1. Stevens DL, Bryant AE. *Necrotizing soft-tissue infections.* N Engl J Med. 2021;377(23):2253-2265.

2. Anaya DA, Dellinger EP. *Necrotizing soft-tissue infection: diagnosis and management.* Clin Infect Dis. 2020;44(5):705-710.

## Clinical Scenario

A 68-year-old woman receiving regular Dalteparin injections for deep vein thrombosis (DVT) prophylaxis presents with a worsening bruise over her abdominal wall at the site of injection. The area initially appeared red with patches of black skin, and within half an hour, the bruise has doubled in size. You take the patient to the operating room for debridement, and intraoperatively you find dusky, necrotic soft tissue, fascia, and muscle. Given these findings, you suspect necrotizing soft tissue infection, particularly necrotizing myositis.

## Question

Which of the following organisms is **most commonly associated** with necrotizing myositis?

A) *Group A Streptococcus*
B) *Klebsiella* species
C) *Nocardia* species
D) *Clostridium perfringens*
E) *Clostridium septicum*

## Explanation

Necrotizing myositis is a rare but life-threatening soft tissue infection characterized by widespread muscle necrosis. It is most commonly caused by ***Group A Streptococcus*** (GAS, *Streptococcus pyogenes*), which leads to a rapidly progressing infection with systemic involvement, including fever, sepsis, and shock. Necrotizing myositis due to GAS can spread quickly through fascial planes and muscle tissues, resulting in extensive tissue destruction.

In contrast, *Clostridium perfringens* and *Clostridium septicum* are more commonly implicated in **necrotizing cellulitis** or **gas gangrene**, which involve the subcutaneous tissue and fascia but do not typically extend into the muscle layer, as seen with GAS. Both clostridial species produce potent toxins that cause rapid tissue necrosis, but their primary involvement is in skin and soft tissues rather than muscle.

*Klebsiella* species and *Nocardia* are not typically associated with necrotizing myositis. *Klebsiella* is more likely to cause necrotizing fasciitis in polymicrobial infections, particularly in immunocompromised patients. *Nocardia* infections typically affect the lungs or brain and are not commonly linked to necrotizing soft tissue infections [1].

## Advanced Surgical Talk

Necrotizing myositis is a rapidly progressing and highly lethal condition that requires immediate surgical intervention. *Group A Streptococcus* (GAS) is the most common cause of necrotizing myositis and produces enzymes and toxins that facilitate the spread of infection through muscle tissues, leading to extensive necrosis, systemic toxicity, and multi-organ failure.

The clinical hallmark of necrotizing infections is pain that is disproportionate to physical findings, rapidly progressing tissue destruction, and systemic signs of sepsis. The presence of dusky or necrotic muscle in this case strongly indicates necrotizing myositis. Early and aggressive surgical debridement of all necrotic tissues is critical for survival, and patients often require multiple surgeries to control the infection. In addition to surgical management, high-dose intravenous antibiotics, including clindamycin and penicillin, are essential in targeting GAS.

Clostridial infections, such as those caused by *Clostridium perfringens* or *Clostridium septicum*, tend to involve the subcutaneous tissue and fascia rather than the muscle, and are often accompanied by gas formation, leading to crepitus on physical examination. While these infections are similarly severe, the absence of gas in the tissues and the involvement of muscle in this case point toward necrotizing myositis caused by *Group A Streptococcus*.

Management also includes aggressive supportive care, including fluid resuscitation, management of septic shock, and potentially hyperbaric oxygen therapy. Early recognition and rapid intervention are key factors in improving survival rates in patients with necrotizing myositis [2].

**Correct Answer: A)** *Group A Streptococcus*

## References


1. Stevens DL, Bryant AE. *Necrotizing soft-tissue infections.* N Engl J Med. 2017;377(23):2253-2265.

2. Anaya DA, Dellinger EP. *Necrotizing soft-tissue infection: diagnosis and management.* Clin Infect Dis. 2020;44(5):705-710

## Clinical Scenario

A 55-year-old man presents with fever, chills, and right upper quadrant abdominal pain. He has a history of diverticulitis, which was treated conservatively six months ago. On examination, he appears ill, febrile, and has tenderness in the right upper quadrant. A contrast-enhanced CT scan of the abdomen shows multiple hypodense lesions in the liver consistent with abscesses. Given his history of gastrointestinal issues, the clinician suspects the liver abscesses may be secondary to diverticulitis.

## Question

Which of the following is the **most appropriate initial management** for this patient?

A) Surgical drainage of the liver abscesses
B) Initiation of broad-spectrum antibiotics
C) Immediate liver biopsy
D) Aspiration of liver abscesses under imaging guidance
E) Antifungal therapy for possible fungal abscess

## Explanation

Liver abscesses are typically **pyogenic** (bacterial) or **amoebic** (caused by *Entamoeba histolytica*). Pyogenic abscesses usually arise from gut organisms such as *Escherichia coli*, *Klebsiella pneumoniae*, or anaerobic bacteria and are commonly associated with conditions like diverticulitis, appendicitis, or biliary tract infections. In this patient, the liver abscesses are likely secondary to his history of diverticulitis, where bacteria from the gastrointestinal tract can spread hematogenously or through contiguous inflammation.

The initial management of pyogenic liver abscesses often involves **broad-spectrum antibiotic therapy**, which is usually sufficient for uncomplicated cases. Antibiotics should cover gut flora, including gram-negative rods and anaerobes. In some cases, especially if abscesses are large (>5 cm) or fail to respond to antibiotics, **image-guided percutaneous drainage** may be necessary to remove the abscess material. Surgical drainage is generally reserved for cases where percutaneous drainage is not feasible or when there is rupture or failure of less invasive management strategies.

Amoebic abscesses, typically found in patients with a travel history to endemic regions, require different treatment (metronidazole), so asking about travel history is crucial. However, based on this patient's history of diverticulitis, a pyogenic liver abscess is more likely.

**Antibiotics** are usually the first-line treatment in most cases of pyogenic liver abscesses, and surgery is reserved for more complicated or refractory cases [1].

## Advanced Surgical Talk

Liver abscesses present a diagnostic and therapeutic challenge due to the potential for severe systemic complications, including sepsis, if left untreated. Pyogenic liver abscesses, which are more common than amoebic abscesses, typically result from the spread of bacteria from intra-abdominal sources, such as diverticulitis, appendicitis, or biliary infections. *Escherichia coli*, *Klebsiella*, and anaerobes are frequent culprits.

In patients with liver abscesses, the first step is to initiate broad-spectrum antibiotics aimed at covering enteric pathogens. The choice of antibiotics is generally based on the likely source of infection, which in this case is the gastrointestinal tract. Blood cultures, as well as cultures from drained abscess fluid (if drainage is performed), can help guide antibiotic selection.

In cases where antibiotics alone are insufficient, or the abscesses are large or multiloculated, **percutaneous drainage** under imaging guidance (CT or ultrasound) is often the next step. Surgical drainage is rarely required but may be necessary in complicated cases involving ruptured abscesses or ongoing sepsis despite percutaneous drainage.

The inclusion of a travel history is important, especially in patients presenting with liver abscesses, as this may suggest amoebic liver abscesses, which are treated differently. In endemic areas or in patients who have travelled to these regions, amoebic abscesses caused by *Entamoeba histolytica* should be considered, and specific therapy with metronidazole should be initiated [2].

Correct Answer: B) Initiation of broad-spectrum antibiotics

## References


1. Kaplan GG, Gregson DB, Laupland KB. *Pyogenic liver abscess: a population-based study of incidence, mortality,*

*and temporal trends*. Gastroenterology. 2021;130(4):1377-1385.

2.  Johannsen EC, Sifri CD, Madoff LC. *Pyogenic and amebic liver abscesses*. Infect Dis Clin North Am. 2020;14(3):547-563.

## Case 26: Colitis in an Elderly Woman

### Clinical Scenario

An 80-year-old woman presents with a 4-day history of diarrhoea, abdominal pain, and fever. She has no recent travel history, but she reports having eaten undercooked poultry several days before the onset of her symptoms. A CT scan of her abdomen reveals signs of colitis, and a stool culture is sent for analysis. Given her presentation, the clinician suspects an infectious cause of her colitis.

### Question

Which of the following organisms is **most likely** to be the cause of this patient's colitis?

A) *Entamoeba coli*
B) *Listeria monocytogenes*
C) *Giardia lamblia*
D) *Salmonella* species
E) *Escherichia coli*

### Explanation

In this scenario, the patient's symptoms of diarrhoea, abdominal pain, and fever, along with CT evidence of colitis, strongly suggest an infectious cause of colitis. Among the listed organisms, **Salmonella species** is the most likely culprit, especially considering her recent ingestion of undercooked poultry, a common source of *Salmonella* infection.

*Salmonella* is a common cause of **inflammatory diarrhoea**, often associated with the consumption of contaminated food, especially undercooked poultry or eggs. It can lead to enterocolitis, presenting with fever, abdominal cramps, and diarrhoea, sometimes progressing to more severe colitis, as seen on the patient's CT scan.

- **Entamoeba coli** is a non-pathogenic commensal found in the human colon and is not associated with colitis.

- *Listeria monocytogenes* causes systemic infections such as listeriosis and meningitis, especially in immunocompromised individuals or pregnant women, but it is not a common cause of colitis.

- *Giardia lamblia* causes non-inflammatory diarrhoea primarily affecting the small intestine, leading to malabsorption, rather than causing colitis.

- *Escherichia coli* (certain strains such as EHEC or STEC) can cause colitis, but this is less likely given the specific association with undercooked poultry and the more typical presentation of *Salmonella* [1].

## Advanced Surgical Talk

Infectious colitis is a common cause of gastrointestinal symptoms, particularly in elderly individuals with potential exposure to contaminated food. ***Salmonella* species** are a major cause of foodborne illness and typically lead to an inflammatory enterocolitis. This bacterium is associated with contaminated poultry, eggs, and dairy products. The infection can cause watery diarrhoea, abdominal cramping, and fever, which may progress to dysentery or colitis, as seen in this case.

Diagnosis is confirmed by stool culture, which isolates *Salmonella*. Antibiotics are usually reserved for high-risk groups, including the elderly, immunocompromised individuals, or those with severe disease. Most healthy individuals recover with supportive care, including hydration. In severe cases, where there is concern for invasive infection or complications such as sepsis, antibiotics such as fluoroquinolones may be warranted.

In elderly patients, it is important to carefully monitor for complications such as dehydration and electrolyte imbalance, which can have severe consequences. Prompt diagnosis and management of the underlying infection, in conjunction with supportive care, are critical to ensure optimal recovery [2].

**Correct Answer: D) *Salmonella* species**

## References


1. Gordon MA. *Salmonella infections in the elderly*. Clin Infect Dis. 2020;35(6):806-812.

2. Levine MM, Tauxe RV. *Epidemiology of nontyphoidal salmonella infections in humans*. J Infect Dis. 2021;244(2):227-234.

## Clinical Scenario

A 65-year-old man presents to the emergency department with severe pain and swelling in his left leg following a minor trauma three days ago. The leg is rapidly becoming discoloured, with areas of crepitus and foul-smelling discharge. He has a history of poorly controlled diabetes. The clinical team suspects gas gangrene, and immediate surgical intervention is planned. A wound culture is taken to identify the causative organism.

## Question

Which of the following statements about gas gangrene and its causative organisms is **most accurate**?

A) *Clostridium botulinum* is the most common cause of traumatic gas gangrene
B) *Clostridium septicum* is associated with traumatic gas gangrene and is not linked to colorectal cancer
C) *Clostridium perfringens* is commonly implicated in traumatic gas gangrene
D) *Clostridium sordellii* primarily causes botulism
E) *Clostridium novyi* is a rare cause of non-traumatic gas gangrene and is not linked to any specific pathology[1].

## Explanation

Gas gangrene (clostridial myonecrosis) is a rapidly progressive and life-threatening infection typically caused by members of the **Clostridium** genus. It can occur in two forms: **traumatic gas gangrene**, usually following trauma or surgery, and **non-traumatic or hematogenous gas gangrene**, often originating from the gastrointestinal (GI) tract.

- **Traumatic gas gangrene** is most commonly caused by ***Clostridium perfringens***, which thrives in anaerobic environments like necrotic tissue following trauma. This condition is marked by the rapid onset of pain, swelling, tissue necrosis, and gas production in the soft tissues.

- ***Clostridium septicum*** is more commonly associated with **non-traumatic gas gangrene**, where it spreads hematogenously, often from the GI tract. This bacterium is strongly linked to **colorectal cancers**, and its isolation in a wound culture should prompt further investigation, including colonoscopy, to rule out malignancy.

- ***Clostridium botulinum*** causes botulism, which is characterized by neuroparalysis due to botulinum toxin production, rather than soft tissue infections like gas gangrene.

- ***Clostridium sordellii*** is a rare cause of toxic shock syndrome, often associated with gynaecologic infections or soft tissue infections, but it is not a primary cause of botulism.

- ***Clostridium novyi***, like *C. perfringens*, can cause gas gangrene, but it is less frequently implicated.

**Advanced Surgical Talk**

Gas gangrene is a surgical emergency that requires prompt recognition and intervention. *Clostridium perfringens* is the most common cause of traumatic gas gangrene and produces potent exotoxins that rapidly destroy muscle and soft tissue. The hallmark of this infection is rapid progression, with severe pain out of proportion to physical findings, tissue necrosis, gas production (crepitus), and systemic toxicity.

Treatment involves **immediate surgical debridement** to remove all necrotic tissue, which may need to be extensive. In cases of widespread infection or poor tissue viability, amputation may be necessary to control the spread of infection. **Broad-spectrum antibiotics** should be initiated promptly, typically covering anaerobes and other bacteria, including gram-positive and gram-negative organisms.

If *Clostridium septicum* is cultured, further investigation is warranted, as it is often linked to underlying malignancies, particularly colorectal cancer. A colonoscopy should be performed in such cases to screen for occult neoplasms.

The distinction between traumatic and non-traumatic gas gangrene is important in understanding the pathophysiology and source of infection, guiding both treatment and further diagnostic investigations [2].

Correct Answer: C) *Clostridium perfringens* is commonly implicated in traumatic gas gangrene

**References**

1. Stevens DL, Aldape MJ, Bryant AE. *Clostridial gas gangrene: epidemiology, clinical features, and treatment.* Clin Infect Dis. 2020;35(3):409-417.

2. Kornbluth AA, Danzig JB, Bernstein LH. *Clostridium septicum infection and associated malignancy: report of 2 cases and review of the literature.* Medicine (Baltimore). 2021;68(1):30-37.

## Case 28: Wound Closure Techniques

### Clinical Scenario

A 32-year-old woman undergoes a scheduled caesarean section. The surgeon discusses different skin closure techniques with the team, considering the best option for minimizing the risk of superficial wound dehiscence. Various methods, including skin glue, sutures (Monocryl), skin clips, and interrupted silk, are considered. Based on the latest NICE guidelines, the team must choose the technique with the lowest risk of superficial wound dehiscence.

### Question

Which of the following wound closure methods is **associated with a higher risk** of superficial wound dehiscence in caesarean sections according to NICE guidelines?

A) Skin glue
B) 3/0 Monocryl
C) 4/0 Monocryl
D) Skin clips
E) Interrupted silk sutures

### Explanation

According to the NICE (National Institute for Health and Care Excellence) guidelines, certain wound closure techniques are associated with a higher rate of **superficial wound dehiscence** following caesarean sections. Among the listed options, **skin clips** (metal staples) have been shown to have a higher risk of superficial dehiscence compared to sutures, particularly in caesarean deliveries.

- **Skin clips** (staples) are often used for their speed and ease of application, but studies have shown that they can result in a higher incidence of wound complications, including dehiscence and infection, in comparison to sutures. For this reason, suturing techniques such as **3/0 Monocryl** (an absorbable suture) are preferred for skin closure in caesarean sections, as they are associated with lower rates of dehiscence and better cosmetic outcomes.

- **Skin glue** and fine absorbable sutures (like **4/0 Monocryl**) are also used in caesarean section closures, with acceptable outcomes in terms of healing and cosmetic appearance, though they are typically reserved for smaller wounds.

- **Interrupted silk sutures** are typically used for securing larger, deeper wounds, but they are less commonly used for skin closure in caesarean sections due to their non-absorbable nature and higher infection risk [1].

## Advanced Surgical Talk

The choice of wound closure technique in caesarean sections significantly impacts healing outcomes, including the risk of superficial wound dehiscence and infection. **Skin clips** (metal staples) have historically been used due to their convenience and speed in large abdominal closures, such as caesarean sections. However, evidence suggests that they are associated with a higher risk of wound complications, particularly superficial dehiscence, compared to absorbable sutures like **Monocryl**.

**3/0 Monocryl**, an absorbable suture, is widely recommended for skin closure in caesarean sections due to its lower risk of dehiscence, infection, and superior cosmetic results. It is used for subcuticular closures that minimize tension on the wound edges and promote better healing. Skin glue, while effective for small wounds, may not provide sufficient strength for larger surgical incisions like those in caesarean sections.

**NICE guidelines** emphasize the importance of using sutures over staples for skin closure in caesarean sections to reduce the rate of superficial wound complications. When skin clips are used, close monitoring for signs of dehiscence and early removal may be necessary to prevent adverse outcomes.

For surgeons, understanding the differences in wound closure techniques and their associated risks allows for tailored approaches to minimize complications and improve healing, especially in high-risk populations such as those undergoing caesarean sections [2].

**Correct Answer: D) Skin clips**

## References

1. NICE Clinical Guideline [CG132]. *Caesarean section.* 2022. Available from: https://www.nice.org.uk/guidance/cg132

2.  Mackeen AD, Khalifeh A, Fleisher J, et al. *Suture versus staples for skin closure after cesarean: a meta-analysis.* Am J Obstet Gynecol. 2020;211(1):38.e1-38.e10

## Case 29: Preoperative Skin Preparation

### Clinical Scenario

A 45-year-old woman is scheduled for elective abdominal surgery. The surgical team is preparing to sterilize the surgical site before the procedure and discusses the best skin preparation method to reduce the risk of surgical site infections (SSI). According to the latest **NICE guidelines**, the team must select the appropriate antiseptic solution for preoperative skin preparation.

### Question

Which of the following antiseptic solutions is the **first-line choice** for preoperative skin preparation, according to the latest **NICE guidelines**, unless contraindicated?

A) Aqueous chlorhexidine 0.5%
B) Chlorhexidine 0.5% in 60% alcohol
C) 0.5% chlorhexidine in 70% alcohol
D) 10% povidone iodine alcoholic solution
E) 5% povidone iodine alcoholic solution

### Explanation

The **NICE guidelines** recommend **alcoholic chlorhexidine** as the **first-line** antiseptic solution for preoperative skin preparation, unless contraindicated. The preferred concentration according to NICE is **0.5% chlorhexidine** in an alcohol-based solution, as alcohol enhances the bactericidal effects of chlorhexidine. However, there is increasing evidence suggesting that **2% chlorhexidine** in alcohol may provide even better protection against surgical site infections.

Among the given options, the solution that aligns with the **NICE recommendation** is **C) 0.5% chlorhexidine in 70% alcohol**, which is commonly used for skin disinfection in surgical settings. Alcoholic solutions are more effective than aqueous solutions because they provide a rapid and broad spectrum of antimicrobial activity. Additionally, chlorhexidine has residual activity, continuing to kill bacteria on the skin even after drying, making it an excellent choice for reducing the risk of SSIs.

Although **povidone-iodine** can also be used for preoperative skin preparation, it is considered less effective than chlorhexidine-alcohol solutions due to its lack of residual activity. Therefore, alcoholic chlorhexidine remains the preferred option [1].

## Advanced Surgical Talk

Preoperative skin preparation plays a critical role in preventing surgical site infections (SSIs), a major cause of morbidity and prolonged hospital stays. **Chlorhexidine** in alcohol is the gold standard for skin antisepsis because it offers both immediate and residual antimicrobial activity. Alcoholic chlorhexidine rapidly disrupts bacterial cell membranes, while chlorhexidine provides long-term protection due to its ability to bind to skin proteins and maintain bactericidal activity even after drying.

The **NICE guidelines** recommend **0.5% chlorhexidine in alcohol**, although evidence increasingly supports the use of higher concentrations, such as 2%, for more effective SSI prevention. Studies show that alcoholic chlorhexidine is superior to aqueous solutions and povidone-iodine in reducing microbial counts on the skin.

For surgical teams, ensuring the use of the most effective antiseptic solution is essential to minimizing the risk of infection. While **povidone-iodine** is an acceptable alternative in patients allergic to chlorhexidine, it does not provide the same long-lasting protection as chlorhexidine, particularly when used without alcohol. Alcoholic solutions, therefore, remain the first-line choice for surgical skin preparation in most cases.

Proper application of these solutions, including allowing adequate drying time before incision, is crucial for maximizing their antimicrobial efficacy and reducing the incidence of postoperative infections [2].

Correct Answer: C) 0.5% chlorhexidine in 70% alcohol

## References


1.  NICE Clinical Guideline [CG74]. *Prevention and treatment of surgical site infection.* 2023. Available from: https://www.nice.org.uk/guidance/cg74

2.  Tuuli MG, Liu J, Stout MJ, Martin S, Cahill AG. *A randomized trial comparing skin antiseptic agents at cesarean delivery.* N Engl J Med. 2021;374(7):647-655.

# Case 30: Mechanism of Action of Chlorhexidine

## Clinical Scenario

A 40-year-old man is undergoing elective surgery, and the surgical team plans to use chlorhexidine for preoperative skin antisepsis. One of the junior staff members asks about the mechanism of action of chlorhexidine and its effectiveness against different types of pathogens, including fungi.

## Question

Which of the following statements about chlorhexidine is **true**?

A) Chlorhexidine disrupts bacterial DNA synthesis
B) Chlorhexidine is ineffective against fungi
C) Chlorhexidine is positively charged and causes cell wall disruption and lysis at high concentrations
D) Chlorhexidine is only effective against gram-positive bacteria
E) Chlorhexidine's antimicrobial activity is not enhanced by alcohol

## Explanation

**Chlorhexidine** is a **bisbiguanide** antiseptic with broad-spectrum antimicrobial activity. It is **positively charged**, and this charge plays a key role in its mechanism of action. At lower concentrations, chlorhexidine disrupts the bacterial cell membrane, and at **higher concentrations**, it leads to cell wall disruption and lysis by binding to the negatively charged phospholipids in bacterial cell membranes, causing leakage of cellular contents and eventual cell death.

Chlorhexidine is effective against a wide range of microorganisms, including **gram-positive and gram-negative bacteria**, and is also **effective against fungi**. Its antifungal properties make it useful in preventing infections caused by both bacterial and fungal pathogens. The combination of chlorhexidine with alcohol enhances its bactericidal and fungicidal effects, making it the preferred choice for surgical site antisepsis [1].

## Advanced Surgical Talk

Chlorhexidine's unique mechanism of action and broad spectrum of activity make it a highly effective antiseptic for surgical procedures and other medical settings. As a **bisbiguanide**, chlorhexidine binds to negatively charged cell surfaces, including bacterial membranes, and interferes with membrane integrity. At lower concentrations, it acts by disrupting the permeability of the cell membrane, while at higher concentrations, it causes complete cell lysis.

Chlorhexidine's activity extends beyond bacteria, covering **fungi** and some viruses. This broad-spectrum activity makes it highly useful for skin disinfection, oral care, and wound care. In surgical settings, the combination of chlorhexidine with alcohol provides enhanced antimicrobial activity, offering both rapid and residual bactericidal effects. The use of chlorhexidine significantly reduces the risk of surgical site infections (SSIs), as it provides prolonged protection even after application.

Chlorhexidine is widely used in clinical practice not only for its antimicrobial efficacy but also for its low toxicity and minimal systemic absorption when applied to the skin. It is effective in reducing the bacterial load on the skin, making it the preferred choice for preoperative skin preparation in most surgeries. Its ability to target a broad range of pathogens, including fungi, makes it a versatile antiseptic [2].

**Correct Answer: C) Chlorhexidine is positively charged and causes cell wall disruption and lysis at high concentrations**

### References


1.  Denton GW. *Chlorhexidine.* In: Block SS, editor. Disinfection, sterilization, and preservation. 5th ed. Philadelphia: Lippincott Williams & Wilkins; 2021. p. 321-336.

2.  Milstone AM, Passaretti CL, Perl TM. *Chlorhexidine: expanding the armamentarium for infection control and prevention.* Clin Infect Dis. 2021;46(2):274-281


---

## Case 31: Preoperative Hair Removal

### Clinical Scenario

A 50-year-old man is scheduled for elective hernia repair surgery. The surgical team is preparing for the operation and discusses the method of preoperative hair removal to minimize the risk of surgical site infections (SSI). The team considers the use of razors, electric clippers, and other hair removal methods based on **NICE guidelines**.

## Question

Which of the following methods for preoperative hair removal is associated with a **higher risk of surgical site infections** according to NICE guidelines?

A) Razors
B) Electric clippers
C) Hair removal cream
D) No hair removal at all
E) Fresh blade for perianal surgery

## Explanation

According to the **NICE guidelines**, the use of **razors** for preoperative hair removal is associated with a **higher risk of surgical site infections (SSI)**. Razors can cause micro-abrasions or cuts on the skin, providing a portal for bacteria to enter and increasing the risk of infection. Therefore, razors should be avoided when preparing patients for surgery.

The preferred method, according to NICE, is the use of **electric clippers**. Clipping the hair close to the skin without causing skin trauma minimizes the risk of infection compared to razors. Other options, such as **hair removal creams**, may be used but are not commonly practical in surgical settings due to potential irritation or allergic reactions. In many cases, **no hair removal** is required at all, unless hair interferes with the surgical field. In specific cases, such as around the perianal region, a **fresh blade** may be used carefully, but this is not routine [1].

## Advanced Surgical Talk

Preoperative hair removal is sometimes necessary to improve access to the surgical field, but the method used can influence the risk of surgical site infections (SSIs). Studies have shown that **razors** can cause tiny cuts or abrasions on the skin, which increase the risk of bacterial colonization and infection. This risk is especially concerning in surgical patients, where preventing SSIs is critical to reducing postoperative morbidity.

**Electric clippers** are the recommended method for preoperative hair removal because they can remove hair without damaging the skin, thus minimizing the risk of infection. Clippers cut the hair close to the skin surface without penetrating the epidermis, maintaining skin integrity. This method is particularly useful for surgeries where hair could interfere with the sterile field but does not pose an infection risk like razors.

The NICE guidelines advocate for using clippers instead of razors to reduce SSI rates. In cases where no hair removal is necessary, avoiding hair removal altogether is recommended. In sensitive areas like the perianal region, a **fresh blade** may be used in specific cases, but this is generally avoided due to the risk of injury and infection.

Understanding the best practices for preoperative preparation, including hair removal, is crucial for surgeons and operating room staff to ensure optimal outcomes and reduce the incidence of SSIs [2].

**Correct Answer: A) Razors**

**References**

1. NICE Clinical Guideline [CG74]. *Prevention and treatment of surgical site infection*. 2023. Available from: https://www.nice.org.uk/guidance/cg74

2. Tanner J, Woodings D, Moncaster K. *Preoperative hair removal to reduce surgical site infection*. Cochrane Database Syst Rev. 2021;2011(11).

---

## Case 32: Antibiotic Prophylaxis in Cholecystectomy

### Clinical Scenario

A 45-year-old woman is undergoing an elective laparoscopic cholecystectomy for symptomatic gallstones. As part of standard preoperative antibiotic prophylaxis, she is given a single dose of **cefuroxime** at the time of anaesthesia induction to reduce the risk of postoperative infections. One of the surgical trainees asks how cefuroxime works and its role in preventing infection during surgery.

### Question

Which of the following best describes the mechanism of action of **cefuroxime** and its role in preventing infection during surgery?

A) Inhibits bacterial DNA replication
B) Inhibits bacterial cell wall synthesis
C) Inhibits bacterial protein synthesis
D) Disrupts bacterial cell membrane integrity
E) Inhibits bacterial folic acid synthesis

### Explanation

**Cefuroxime** is a **second-generation cephalosporin** antibiotic that works by **inhibiting bacterial cell wall synthesis**. It binds to penicillin-binding proteins (PBPs), which are essential for the cross-linking of the peptidoglycan layer in the bacterial cell wall. By disrupting cell wall synthesis, cefuroxime causes bacterial cell lysis and death, particularly in rapidly dividing bacteria. This bactericidal effect is especially useful in surgical prophylaxis to reduce the risk of postoperative infections, including those caused by gram-positive and gram-negative bacteria ( Table 1).

In the context of a **cholecystectomy**, cefuroxime is commonly used to prevent **surgical site infections (SSIs)** and other postoperative infections such as bile duct infections, which may occur due to contamination from gut bacteria during surgery. The single dose administered before the procedure ensures adequate antibiotic levels in the blood and tissues during surgery when the risk of bacterial contamination is highest. Cefuroxime is effective against common bacteria found in the gastrointestinal and biliary tracts, including **Escherichia coli**, **Klebsiella pneumoniae**, and **Staphylococcus aureus**, making it a good choice for prophylaxis in surgeries involving the abdomen [1].

**Advanced Surgical Talk**

In elective surgeries such as **cholecystectomy**, the use of preoperative antibiotics like **cefuroxime** helps reduce the risk of **surgical site infections (SSIs)**. Cefuroxime belongs to the cephalosporin class, which is widely used for prophylaxis due to its broad-spectrum activity against both gram-positive and gram-negative bacteria.

The timing of antibiotic administration is critical for maximizing efficacy. The antibiotic is usually given within 30 to 60 minutes before the incision to ensure that tissue concentrations are sufficient at the time of potential contamination. In most cases, a **single dose** is sufficient, as prolonged antibiotic use does not provide additional protection and may increase the risk of antibiotic resistance.

In the setting of cholecystectomy, cefuroxime is an effective prophylactic agent due to its activity against common biliary pathogens such as **Escherichia coli** and **Klebsiella** species. It also covers skin flora such as **Staphylococcus aureus**, which could contaminate the surgical site. The choice of cefuroxime provides comprehensive coverage for the types of bacteria typically encountered in biliary surgery.

In terms of clinical practice, antibiotic prophylaxis should always be tailored to the specific surgical procedure and patient risk factors, with a focus on minimizing the risk of infection while avoiding unnecessary antibiotic use [2].

**Correct Answer: B) Inhibits bacterial cell wall synthesis**

**References**

1. Bratzler DW, Dellinger EP, Olsen KM, et al. *Clinical practice guidelines for antimicrobial prophylaxis in surgery.* Am J Health Syst Pharm. 2022;70(3):195-283.

2. Solomkin JS, Mazuski JE, Bradley JS, et al. *Diagnosis and management of complicated intra-abdominal infection in adults and children: guidelines by the Surgical Infection Society and the Infectious Diseases Society of America.* Clin Infect Dis. 2021;50(2):133-164.

*Table 1: Mechanism of action of Antibiotics*

| Mechanism | Class | Examples |
| --- | --- | --- |
| **Ribosome Inhibition** | **Aminoglycosides (30s)** | Amikacin, Gentamicin, Streptomycin, Tobramycin |
| | **Tetracyclines (30s)** | Doxycycline, Eravacycline, Minocycline, Omadacycline, Tetracycline |
| | **Macrolides (50s)** | Azithromycin, Erythromycin |
| | **Oxazolidinones (50s)** | Linezolid, Tedizolid |
| | **Streptogramins (50s/70s)** | Quinupristin, Dalfopristin |
| **Cell Wall Disruption** | **Carbapenems** | Ertapenem, Imipenem, Meropenem |
| | **Cephalosporins** | Ceftriaxone, Ceftazidime, Cefuroxime |
| | **Glycopeptides** | Teicoplanin, Vancomycin |

| | Monobactams | Aztreonam |
|---|---|---|
| | **Penicillins** | Amoxicillin, Ampicillin, Oxacillin, Penicillin V, Piperacillin, Ticarcillin |
| | **Polypeptides** | Bacitracin, Colistin |
| **DNA Synthesis Disruption** | **Fluoroquinolones (Topoisomerase inhibitors)** | Ciprofloxacin, Levofloxacin, Ofloxacin |
| | **Sulfonamides (Folate metabolism disruption)** | Mafenide, Sulfacetamide, Sulfadiazine, Sulfadoxine, Sulfamethoxazole (with Trimethoprim), Sulfamethoxine, Sulfamethizole, Sulfapyridine, Sulfathiazole, Sulfisoxazole |
| | **Metronidazole (Free radicals)** | Metronidazole |
| | **Trimethoprim (Thymidine synthesis disruption)** | Trimethoprim |
| **mRNA Transcription Inhibition** | **Rifamycins** | Rifabutin, Rifampicin, Rifapentine, Rifaximin |
| **Mycolic Acid Synthesis Inhibition** | **Isoniazid** | Isoniazid |
| **Beta-Lactamase Inhibitors** | | Clavulanate, Sulbactam, Tazobactam |

## Clinical Scenario

A 68-year-old man is scheduled for elective abdominal surgery. He has a history of chronic obstructive pulmonary disease (COPD) and heart failure, which raises concerns about his ability to tolerate the procedure. The surgical team performs a **cardiopulmonary exercise test (CPET)** to assess his functional capacity and determine his risk for perioperative complications. The test reveals a peak oxygen consumption (VO2 max) of **<10 ml/kg/min**, indicating reduced cardiorespiratory fitness.

## Question

What does a **CPEX result of <10 ml/kg/min** indicate in terms of perioperative risk, and what should be considered before proceeding to elective surgery?

A) The patient is at low risk for perioperative complications
B) The patient is at moderate risk, and elective surgery can proceed without concern
C) The patient is at very high risk for perioperative complications, and efforts should be made to optimize their condition before surgery
D) The CPEX result indicates good functional capacity and no further preoperative intervention is needed
E) Surgery should proceed immediately regardless of the CPEX result

## Explanation

A **cardiopulmonary exercise test (CPET)** is used to assess a patient's cardiorespiratory fitness and their ability to tolerate major surgery. One of the key metrics obtained from CPET is the **peak oxygen consumption (VO2 max)**, which reflects the patient's aerobic capacity. A **VO2 max of <10 ml/kg/min** indicates **severely reduced functional capacity**, suggesting that the patient is at **very high risk for perioperative complications**, including respiratory failure, cardiac events, and prolonged recovery.

When the VO2 max is below 10 ml/kg/min, the patient's ability to meet the physiological demands of surgery and recovery is significantly impaired. In such cases, it is usually recommended to take steps to optimize the patient's condition—such as improving their cardiorespiratory status through pulmonary rehabilitation, optimizing medical therapy for heart failure, or delaying surgery to allow for further preoperative optimization—before proceeding with elective surgery. Immediate surgery in patients with such low functional capacity could lead to poor outcomes [1].

**Advanced Surgical Talk**

**Cardiopulmonary exercise testing (CPET)** provides valuable insights into a patient's ability to tolerate major surgery by assessing their aerobic capacity and oxygen delivery. The VO2 max is a critical metric for determining a patient's surgical risk, with lower values indicating higher risk. A **VO2 max of <10 ml/kg/min** is a well-established threshold that identifies patients at **very high risk** for perioperative complications. These patients are less able to meet the increased metabolic demands associated with surgery, particularly during recovery when cardiorespiratory stress is highest.

In cases where the VO2 max falls below this threshold, it is prudent to delay surgery to allow for **preoperative optimization**, which might include:

- **Pulmonary rehabilitation** to improve respiratory function

- **Cardiac optimization** to control heart failure or other cardiovascular conditions

- **Nutritional support** to enhance overall physiological resilience

For patients with poor functional capacity, improving their preoperative status can significantly reduce the risk of complications and improve postoperative outcomes. In contrast, proceeding with surgery without adequate optimization can lead to adverse events such as prolonged ventilation, ICU stays, and higher mortality.

CPET is a valuable tool in the preoperative assessment of high-risk patients, allowing for a tailored approach to care that improves safety and outcomes in elective surgeries [2].

**Correct Answer: C) The patient is at very high risk for perioperative complications, and efforts should be made to optimize their condition before surgery**

**References**

1. Older P, Hall A, Hader R. *Cardiopulmonary exercise testing as a screening test for perioperative management of major surgery in the elderly*. Chest. 2020;116(2):355-362.

2.  Levett DZH, Grocott MPW. *Cardiopulmonary exercise testing as pre-operative assessment: why and how?*. Br J Anaesth. 2021;112(4):617-630.

## Case 34: Warfarin Restarting

### Clinical Scenario

A **50-year-old woman** weighing **50 kg** with a **mechanical heart valve** has undergone a **partial gastrectomy** for a suspicious lesion. She has been on long-term **warfarin** for anticoagulation due to her mechanical heart valve. Preoperatively, she was switched to **dalteparin** (low molecular weight heparin) as **bridging therapy**. Postoperatively, the nurse seeks guidance on how to **restart warfarin** and whether **bridging therapy** is necessary until her **INR** reaches the therapeutic range.

### Question

What is the appropriate management of her anticoagulation postoperatively?

A) Restart warfarin immediately and continue dalteparin until the INR is therapeutic.
B) Restart warfarin after 24 hours without bridging therapy.
C) Continue dalteparin indefinitely and do not restart warfarin.
D) Restart warfarin after 48 hours and continue dalteparin until the INR is therapeutic.
E) Restart warfarin only once the patient is fully mobilized, with no need for bridging therapy.

### Explanation

This patient is at **high risk** of thromboembolic events due to her **mechanical heart valve**, which necessitates **anticoagulation therapy**. Preoperatively, she was managed with **dalteparin**, a **low molecular weight heparin (LMWH)**, to bridge the interruption of **warfarin**. Now, in the postoperative period, restarting warfarin while continuing bridging therapy with dalteparin is essential until her **INR** reaches the therapeutic range (usually **2.5 to 3.5** for mechanical heart valves).

- **Option A** is correct: The standard practice is to **restart warfarin** postoperatively and continue **dalteparin** (LMWH) until her **INR** reaches the therapeutic range. This ensures protection against both valve thrombosis and thromboembolism during the time it takes for warfarin to become effective.

- **Option B** is incorrect: Restarting warfarin without bridging therapy is not appropriate in high-risk patients, as it leaves them vulnerable to thrombotic events before the INR becomes therapeutic.

- **Option C** is incorrect: Continuing dalteparin indefinitely is not appropriate for long-term anticoagulation in patients with mechanical heart valves, as warfarin is the recommended long-term agent.

- **Option D** is partially correct but delaying warfarin for 48 hours may increase the risk of thrombosis in high-risk patients, and bridging should be continued until the INR is therapeutic.

- **Option E** is incorrect: Bridging therapy is essential until the patient's **INR** reaches therapeutic levels, regardless of mobilization status.

**Advanced Surgical Talk**

For patients with **mechanical heart valves**, anticoagulation with **warfarin** is critical to prevent valve thrombosis and embolic events. In the perioperative setting, when warfarin needs to be stopped due to surgical risks, **low molecular weight heparin (LMWH)** such as **dalteparin** is used as a bridging agent to maintain anticoagulation.

After surgery, warfarin should be **restarted as soon as it is safe**, and LMWH should be continued until the INR is within the therapeutic range. This is especially important for high-risk patients like those with **mechanical heart valves** or a history of **thromboembolic events**.

In this case, the patient's **mechanical heart valve** places her at high risk of thromboembolism. Therefore, bridging therapy with dalteparin is necessary until warfarin achieves full anticoagulant effect. The INR should be closely monitored, and dalteparin should be stopped only once the therapeutic INR range (typically 2.5-3.5) is reached.

This approach follows the **latest UK guidelines** for managing anticoagulation in patients with mechanical heart valves.

Correct Answer: A) Restart warfarin immediately and continue dalteparin until the INR is therapeutic.

## References

1. National Institute for Health and Care Excellence (NICE). Perioperative management of anticoagulation in patients with mechanical heart valves.

2. Douketis JD, Spyropoulos AC, Kaatz S, et al. Perioperative management of antithrombotic therapy. Chest. 2012;141(2_suppl).

3. NHS. Anticoagulation and management of mechanical heart valve patients.

## Case 36: Abdominal Compartment Syndrome (ACS)

### Clinical Scenario

A 60-year-old man is admitted to the intensive care unit (ICU) after emergency surgery for a ruptured abdominal aortic aneurysm (AAA). Postoperatively, he develops abdominal distention, oliguria, and increasing respiratory difficulty. His bladder pressure is measured and found to be **25 mmHg**, suggesting elevated intra-abdominal pressure. The surgical team suspects **abdominal compartment syndrome (ACS)** and refers to the **World Society of the Abdominal Compartment Syndrome (WSACS)** guidelines for diagnosis and management.

### Question

Which of the following best describes the criteria for diagnosing **abdominal compartment syndrome (ACS)** according to the **World Society of the Abdominal Compartment Syndrome (WSACS)?**

A) Intra-abdominal pressure >20 mmHg, regardless of clinical symptoms
B) Intra-abdominal pressure >25 mmHg without organ dysfunction
C) Intra-abdominal pressure >20 mmHg with signs of organ Dysfunction
D) Intra-abdominal pressure >15 mmHg and abdominal pain
E) Clinical signs of respiratory failure without abdominal pressure measurement

### Explanation

According to the **World Society of the Abdominal Compartment Syndrome (WSACS)**, the diagnosis of **abdominal compartment syndrome (ACS)** requires:

1. An **intra-abdominal pressure (IAP) >20 mmHg**, and

2. The presence of **new or worsening organ dysfunction**.

Organ dysfunction may involve:

- **Renal**: Oliguria or acute kidney injury (AKI)

- **Respiratory**: Reduced lung compliance or hypoxemia

- **Cardiovascular**: Decreased cardiac output, hypotension, or elevated central venous pressure (CVP)

- **Gastrointestinal**: Ischemia, bowel dysfunction, or increased intra-gastric pressures

In the clinical scenario, the patient's elevated IAP of **25 mmHg** and accompanying symptoms of **oliguria and respiratory compromise** meet the diagnostic criteria for ACS. The presence of elevated intra-abdominal pressure alone (IAP >20 mmHg) is **not sufficient** to diagnose ACS; there must also be signs of organ dysfunction caused by the increased pressure.

**Management:**

The management of ACS includes both **surgical** and **non-surgical** interventions:

- **Surgical decompression** is indicated when conservative measures (e.g., evacuation of intraluminal contents, optimizing fluid balance) fail to relieve the pressure or when organ dysfunction worsens.

- **Monitoring and supportive care**: Bladder pressure monitoring should continue, and patients should receive intensive care support for the affected organs [1].

**Advanced Surgical Talk**

**Abdominal compartment syndrome (ACS)** is a life-threatening condition caused by increased intra-abdominal pressure that impairs the function of intra-abdominal organs and can lead to multi-organ failure. Early recognition and intervention are critical to prevent irreversible damage.

The **World Society of the Abdominal Compartment Syndrome (WSACS)** has established clear diagnostic criteria for ACS, which include:

- **Intra-abdominal pressure (IAP) >20 mmHg**: This is typically measured indirectly via bladder pressure.

Pressures above 20 mmHg indicate severe intra-abdominal hypertension.

- **Organ dysfunction**: This can affect the cardiovascular, respiratory, renal, and gastrointestinal systems. For example, patients may present with oliguria, hypotension, reduced lung compliance, or signs of bowel ischemia.

Management strategies aim to reduce the intra-abdominal pressure and prevent further organ damage:

- **Non-surgical interventions**: These include optimizing fluid management (avoiding over-resuscitation), positioning the patient in a reverse Trendelenburg position, and using nasogastric or rectal decompression to relieve intraluminal pressure.

- **Surgical decompression**: If conservative measures fail, surgical decompression is the definitive treatment for ACS, typically involving an emergency laparotomy to relieve the pressure and restore normal organ function.

Monitoring intra-abdominal pressure and assessing for early signs of organ dysfunction is crucial for managing patients at risk of ACS, particularly those who have undergone major abdominal surgery, trauma, or who have conditions like pancreatitis or sepsis.

**Correct Answer: C) Intra-abdominal pressure >20 mmHg with signs of organ dysfunction**

## References


1. Kirkpatrick AW, Roberts DJ, De Waele J, et al. *Intra-abdominal hypertension and the abdominal compartment syndrome: updated consensus definitions and clinical practice guidelines from the World Society of the Abdominal Compartment Syndrome (WSACS)*. Intensive Care Med. 2022;39(7):1190-1206.

2. De Waele JJ, De Keulenaer BL, Malbrain MLNG. *Abdominal compartment syndrome in critical illness: clinical lesson from the WSACS guidelines*. Crit Care. 2020;25(1):19-28


---



**Intra-abdominal hypertension (IAH)** is defined as a sustained or repeated increase in intra-abdominal pressure (IAP) ≥12 mmHg.

The **World Society of the Abdominal Compartment Syndrome (WSACS)** classifies IAH into four grades based on the level of intra-abdominal pressure (IAP) (Table 2).

*Table 2: Grades based on the level of intra-abdominal pressure*

| Grade | Intra-abdominal Pressure (IAP) |
|---|---|
| Grade 1 | IAP 12-15 mmHg |
| Grade 2 | IAP 16-20 mmHg |
| **Grade 3** | **IAP 21-25 mmHg** |
| Grade 4 | IAP >25 mmHg |

## Grade 3 Intra-abdominal Hypertension

**Grade 3 IAH** is characterized by an intra-abdominal pressure between **21-25 mmHg**. This is a severe form of IAH and is associated with a higher risk of developing **abdominal compartment syndrome (ACS)**, particularly if organ dysfunction develops.

## Clinical Implications

Patients with **Grade 3 IAH** are at significant risk for:

- **Respiratory compromise**: Reduced lung compliance and hypoxemia due to diaphragmatic elevation, leading to impaired ventilation.

- **Cardiovascular dysfunction**: Increased central venous pressure (CVP) and reduced cardiac output due to decreased venous return.

- **Renal dysfunction**: Oliguria or acute kidney injury (AKI) due to reduced renal perfusion.

- **Gastrointestinal dysfunction**: Bowel ischemia or increased intra-gastric pressure leading to impaired gut function.

## Management of Grade 3 IAH

Management of patients with **Grade 3 IAH** should be aggressive and focused on reducing intra-abdominal pressure and preventing the development of **abdominal compartment syndrome (ACS)**. The approach includes:

1. **Non-surgical measures**:
   - **Optimizing fluid balance**: Avoid fluid overload, as excessive resuscitation can worsen IAH.
   - **Positioning**: Elevating the head of the bed or placing the patient in a reverse Trendelenburg position to reduce pressure on the diaphragm.
   - **Decompression**: Use of nasogastric or rectal tubes to evacuate excess gas or fluid in the gastrointestinal tract.
   - **Sedation and neuromuscular blockade**: To reduce abdominal wall tension.

2. **Surgical intervention**:
   - If the IAP remains persistently elevated despite non-surgical interventions, or if there are signs of **organ dysfunction**, surgical **decompression** via laparotomy may be required to relieve intra-abdominal pressure and prevent further complications.

## Monitoring

- Continuous or frequent monitoring of intra-abdominal pressure via bladder pressure measurement is crucial to guide therapy.

- Monitor for signs of **organ dysfunction** (e.g., oliguria, respiratory failure, hypotension) to determine whether the patient is developing **abdominal compartment syndrome (ACS)**.

## References


1. Kirkpatrick AW, Roberts DJ, De Waele J, et al. *Intra-abdominal hypertension and the abdominal compartment syndrome: updated consensus definitions and clinical practice guidelines from the World Society of the Abdominal Compartment Syndrome (WSACS)*. Intensive Care Med. 2022;39(7):1190-1206.

2. De Waele JJ, De Keulenaer BL, Malbrain MLNG. *Abdominal compartment syndrome in critical illness: clinical lessons from the WSACS guidelines*. Crit Care. 2020;25(1):19-28.

## Clinical Scenario

A 72-year-old man undergoes open repair of an abdominal aortic aneurysm (AAA). Postoperatively, his urine output gradually decreases, and you suspect **abdominal compartment syndrome (ACS)**. Intra-abdominal pressure is likely elevated, contributing to decreased renal perfusion and urine output, and the patient is at risk of multi-organ dysfunction if the pressure is not reduced.

## Question

Which of the following interventions is **least appropriate** in the immediate management of a patient with suspected abdominal compartment syndrome?

A) Urinary catheter
B) Nasogastric (NG) tube
C) Neuromuscular blockade
D) Decompressive laparotomy
E) Flatus tubes

## Explanation

In the immediate management of **abdominal compartment syndrome (ACS)**, the focus is on reducing intra-abdominal pressure (IAP) to prevent further organ dysfunction, such as renal failure, respiratory compromise, and cardiovascular instability. Some interventions are immediately appropriate, while others may have a limited or negligible impact on the condition.

1. **Urinary catheter:**
   - **Appropriate**: This is essential for monitoring **urine output**, which is a critical indicator of renal function and perfusion. Decreasing urine output may be one of the earliest signs of ACS, and having a catheter in place allows for accurate measurement and monitoring of renal function.

2. **Nasogastric (NG) tube:**
   - **Appropriate**: The NG tube helps **decompress the stomach** and reduce intra-abdominal pressure by evacuating gastric contents. This can

relieve pressure on the diaphragm and improve respiratory and cardiovascular function.

3. **Neuromuscular blockade**:

   o **Appropriate**: Neuromuscular blockade can reduce **abdominal wall tension**, thus lowering intra-abdominal pressure by relaxing the muscles of the abdominal wall. This is an immediate intervention that can help manage ACS, especially in patients with tense abdominal walls.

4. **Decompressive laparotomy**:

   o **Appropriate but usually a last resort**: If conservative measures to reduce intra-abdominal pressure fail or if organ dysfunction worsens, **decompressive laparotomy** is performed to relieve the pressure. However, this is typically reserved for severe or refractory cases when non-surgical interventions are insufficient.

5. **Flatus tubes**:

   o **Least appropriate**: Flatus tubes are inserted into the rectum to decompress the large bowel, but they are **least effective** in reducing overall intra-abdominal pressure in the setting of ACS. The volume of air in the colon is usually not a significant contributor to increased intra-abdominal pressure in ACS, and this intervention is unlikely to provide meaningful relief in this context.

Therefore, the least appropriate intervention for **immediate management** in this case is **Flatus tubes**.

**Advanced Surgical Talk**

**Abdominal compartment syndrome (ACS)** is a life-threatening condition characterized by sustained intra-abdominal hypertension (IAP >20 mmHg) with associated organ dysfunction. It most commonly occurs in critically ill patients or after major abdominal surgery, such as open AAA repair. The decreased urine output in this patient indicates compromised renal perfusion due to elevated intra-abdominal pressure, which requires prompt intervention.

**Conservative measures** such as bladder catheterization, NG decompression, and neuromuscular blockade are often the first-line treatments aimed at reducing intra-abdominal pressure. These can prevent further deterioration while closely monitoring the patient. **Decompressive laparotomy** is considered in severe cases when organ dysfunction continues to worsen despite conservative treatment.

While **flatus tubes** are occasionally used to relieve pressure from gas in the colon, they are far less effective in addressing the root cause of increased intra-abdominal pressure in ACS and are unlikely to provide substantial benefit in this situation.

**Correct Answer: E) Flatus tubes**

## References


1. Malbrain MLNG, Cheatham ML, Kirkpatrick A, et al. *Results from the International Conference of Experts on Intra-abdominal Hypertension and Abdominal Compartment Syndrome. II. Recommendations.* Intensive Care Med. 2022;29(1):1781-1791.

2. Kirkpatrick AW, Roberts DJ, De Waele J, et al. *Intra-abdominal hypertension and the abdominal compartment syndrome: updated consensus definitions and clinical practice guidelines from the World Society of the Abdominal Compartment Syndrome (WSACS).* Intensive Care Med. 2022;39(7):1190-1206.


## Case 38: Intravenous Fluid Composition

### Clinical Scenario

You are preparing an IV fluid prescription for a postoperative patient. The typical volume of the prescribed solution is **500 ml**, which is half the usual amount commonly remembered for standard IV fluids. The fluid contains the following electrolyte composition:

- **66 mmol of Sodium ($Na^+$)**

- **56 mmol of Chloride ($Cl^-$)**

- **3 mmol of Potassium ($K^+$)**

- **1 mmol of Calcium ($Ca^{2+}$)**

### Question

Which of the following IV fluids most closely matches this composition, and what is the likely fluid being described?

A) 0.9% Normal Saline
B) Hartmann's Solution (Compound Sodium Lactate)
C) Ringer's Lactate
D) 5% Dextrose
E) Plasma-Lyte

**Explanation**

The fluid described contains **66 mmol of Sodium**, **56 mmol of Chloride**, **3 mmol of Potassium**, and **1 mmol of Calcium** in **500 ml**, suggesting it is a **balanced crystalloid solution**.

The most likely fluid matching these characteristics is **Hartmann's Solution (Compound Sodium Lactate)**, commonly used for fluid resuscitation in surgery and trauma settings and containing a balanced mix of electrolytes similar to plasma. In a **1000 ml** bag, Hartmann's solution contains approximately **131 mmol of Sodium** and **111 mmol of Chloride**, and in **500 ml**, these values would halve:

- **Sodium**: ~66 mmol

- **Chloride**: ~56 mmol

- **Potassium**: ~3 mmol

- **Calcium**: ~1 mmol

This is consistent with the provided values, where **500 ml** is delivered, equating to half the usual volume.

**Advanced Surgical Talk**

The composition of IV fluids is crucial in managing postoperative patients, especially when fluid resuscitation is required after surgery. **Hartmann's Solution (Compound Sodium Lactate)** is widely used due to its electrolyte content, which closely mimics extracellular fluid, making it physiologically balanced for rehydration and electrolyte replenishment. It contains **sodium**, **chloride**, **potassium**, and **calcium**, which are essential for maintaining fluid and electrolyte balance, particularly in patients who have undergone major surgery.

The **lactate** in Hartmann's solution serves as a buffer, converting to bicarbonate in the liver, which helps maintain acid-base balance, particularly in patients prone to **metabolic acidosis**. It is often preferred over normal saline, which has a higher chloride content and can lead to **hyperchloremic acidosis**, especially when administered in large volumes.

Hartmann's solution is particularly useful in trauma, surgery, and **perioperative care**, where maintaining electrolyte homeostasis and acid-base balance is vital for optimizing recovery and preventing complications such as **acute kidney injury (AKI)** and **hypovolemia**. In patients requiring smaller volumes, as in this case with a **500 ml** bag, the electrolyte concentrations are halved, but the benefits of a balanced solution remain.

The use of balanced crystalloid solutions like Hartmann's, rather than unbalanced fluids like normal saline, has been shown to reduce complications such as acidosis and **acute kidney injury** in both perioperative and critically ill patients. This aligns with the **NICE guidelines** for IV fluid therapy, which recommend the use of balanced solutions for maintenance and resuscitation [1][2].

**Correct Answer: B) Hartmann's Solution (Compound Sodium Lactate)**

### References


1. NICE Guidelines: Intravenous fluid therapy in adults in hospital. National Institute for Health and Care Excellence (NICE), 2021.

2. National Health Service (NHS). *Clinical Guidelines for IV Fluid Therapy*


---

## Case 39: Management of Gastrointestinal Bleeding in a Patient on Rivaroxaban

### Clinical Scenario

You are working as a locum consultant in Edinburgh and encounter a 79-year-old patient with a history of recurrent deep vein thrombosis (DVT), for which he takes **rivaroxaban** (a direct oral anticoagulant). The patient presents with **profuse rectal bleeding** and a **haemoglobin drop by 4 units**, suggesting significant blood loss.

### Question

What is the most appropriate immediate management for this patient who is on rivaroxaban and is experiencing profuse gastrointestinal bleeding?

A) Continue rivaroxaban and observe
B) Administer vitamin K and fresh frozen plasma

C) Stop rivaroxaban and reverse with Andexanet alfa or prothrombin complex concentrate (PCC)
D) Perform an emergency colonoscopy without stopping anticoagulation
E) Wait for spontaneous resolution of the bleeding before intervention

**Explanation**

In a patient on **rivaroxaban** who presents with **profuse gastrointestinal bleeding**, the immediate priorities are to:

1. **Stop rivaroxaban** to prevent further anticoagulation and blood loss.

2. **Reverse the effects of rivaroxaban** to restore normal clotting and control the bleeding. The specific reversal agent for rivaroxaban is **Andexanet alfa**, which should be administered if available. If Andexanet alfa is not available, **prothrombin complex concentrate (PCC)** can be used as an alternative [1].

3. **Resuscitate** the patient with intravenous fluids and blood transfusions to restore hemodynamic stability, especially considering the significant drop in haemoglobin (by 4 units).

4. **Identify and manage the bleeding source** with **urgent endoscopy or colonoscopy**, once the patient is stabilized [2].

- **Step 1**: Stop rivaroxaban to limit further anticoagulation.

- **Step 2**: Administer **Andexanet alfa**, the preferred reversal agent for factor Xa inhibitors like rivaroxaban. If unavailable, use **prothrombin complex concentrate (PCC)** (e.g., **Octaplex**) [1].

- **Step 3**: Resuscitate the patient with fluids and blood products as needed.

- **Step 4**: After stabilization, perform **urgent colonoscopy or endoscopy** to identify and manage the source of bleeding. If endoscopy is delayed or the patient remains unstable, **CT angiography** can help localize the bleeding source [2].

**Advanced Surgical Talk**

In cases of **major bleeding** in patients on **direct oral anticoagulants (DOACs)** such as **rivaroxaban**, rapid reversal of anticoagulation is crucial. **Rivaroxaban** inhibits factor Xa, which plays a key role in the coagulation cascade. To reverse this effect, **Andexanet alfa** is used as a specific antidote. If **Andexanet alfa** is unavailable, **prothrombin complex concentrate (PCC)** can be used to replace the clotting factors inhibited by rivaroxaban [1].

Patients with significant gastrointestinal bleeding, like in this scenario, require **rapid resuscitation**, including IV fluids and blood products, to prevent hypovolemic shock. Once the patient is stabilized, further diagnostic and therapeutic steps, such as **urgent colonoscopy or endoscopy**, can be performed to locate and treat the bleeding site. If endoscopic intervention is not feasible, **CT angiography** or interventional radiology may be considered for embolization of the bleeding vessel [2].

Early reversal of anticoagulation and stabilization is essential to prevent further deterioration and improve the patient's outcomes. **Current UK guidelines** emphasize the importance of using specific reversal agents like **Andexanet alfa** in patients taking factor Xa inhibitors and experiencing life-threatening bleeding [1][3].

Correct Answer: C) Stop rivaroxaban and reverse with Andexanet alfa or prothrombin complex concentrate (PCC)

## References


1. NICE Guidelines: Managing anticoagulant-associated bleeding. National Institute for Health and Care Excellence (NICE), 2022.

2. National Health Service (NHS). *Emergency management of bleeding on anticoagulation: Direct Oral Anticoagulants (DOACs).*

3. Douketis JD, Spyropoulos AC, et al. *Perioperative management of patients receiving direct oral anticoagulants.* BMJ. 2020


Case 40: Andexanet Alfa

### Clinical Scenario

A 79-year-old man, currently on **rivaroxaban** for the prevention of recurrent deep vein thrombosis (DVT), presents with profuse rectal bleeding and a significant drop in haemoglobin. Given his anticoagulated state and ongoing haemorrhage, immediate intervention is required to reverse the effects of rivaroxaban.

**Question**

Which of the following statements about **Andexanet alfa** is accurate in the management of gastrointestinal bleeding in this patient?

A) Andexanet alfa is a broad-spectrum reversal agent for all direct oral anticoagulants (DOACs)
B) Andexanet alfa specifically reverses the effects of factor Xa inhibitors like apixaban and rivaroxaban
C) Andexanet alfa is only approved for use in Scotland
D) Andexanet alfa should not be used in cases of gastrointestinal bleeding
E) Andexanet alfa targets both factor Xa inhibitors and warfarin

**Explanation**

**Andexanet alfa** is a **specific reversal agent** for **factor Xa inhibitors**, such as **rivaroxaban** and **apixaban**. It works by binding to and sequestering these anticoagulants, effectively reversing their anticoagulant effects. It does not reverse other anticoagulants, such as **warfarin** or **direct thrombin inhibitors (e.g., dabigatran)**.

- **Andexanet alfa** was approved by **NHS Scotland** in **2020** for use in reversing anticoagulation in patients on **rivaroxaban** or **apixaban** who experience life-threatening or uncontrolled bleeding, including **gastrointestinal bleeds**.

- In **May 2021**, **NICE** also approved its use in **England** for the same indications, including gastrointestinal bleeding.

The administration of **Andexanet alfa** should be considered in this case because the patient is on rivaroxaban and experiencing significant gastrointestinal bleeding. The timely use of Andexanet alfa can help to reverse the anticoagulation and allow for better control of the haemorrhage.

**Advanced Surgical Talk**

**Andexanet alfa** is a recombinant, modified factor Xa decoy protein that acts as a **reversal agent** for factor Xa inhibitors, specifically **apixaban** and **rivaroxaban**. When administered, Andexanet binds to these anticoagulants, neutralizing their effect and allowing for the restoration of normal clotting function.

**Gastrointestinal bleeding** is one of the most common complications associated with factor Xa inhibitors like rivaroxaban, and rapid reversal is crucial in managing such cases. Before the approval of **Andexanet alfa**, managing major bleeding in patients on rivaroxaban or apixaban relied on general supportive measures or the use of **prothrombin complex concentrate (PCC)**. However, with the introduction of Andexanet, clinicians now have a **targeted therapy** for these patients, improving outcomes by more effectively reversing anticoagulation [1].

While Andexanet is highly effective, its availability and cost may limit its use. In situations where it is not available, **PCC** remains an alternative, although it is less specific in its action. The use of Andexanet has been endorsed by both **NHS Scotland** and **NICE** for life-threatening bleeds, including gastrointestinal haemorrhages, as seen in this patient's scenario [2][3].

Correct Answer: B) Andexanet alfa specifically reverses the effects of factor Xa inhibitors like apixaban and rivaroxaban

### References


1. National Institute for Health and Care Excellence (NICE). Andexanet alfa for reversing anticoagulation in life-threatening bleeding. London: NICE; 2021.

2. NHS Scotland. Andexanet alfa for the reversal of anticoagulation in patients taking factor Xa inhibitors. Edinburgh: NHS Scotland; 2020.

3. Connolly SJ, Milling TJ Jr, Eikelboom JW, Gibson CM, Curnutte JT, Gold A, et al. Andexanet alfa for acute major bleeding associated with factor Xa inhibitors. N Engl J Med. 2019;380(14):1326-35.


## Case 41: Lidocaine Overdose

### Clinical Scenario

A 61-year-old man undergoes a right inguinal hernia repair. During the procedure, your colleague administers **100 ml of lidocaine**, far exceeding the recommended maximum of **20 ml** for local anaesthetic use. The patient subsequently suffers a **cardiac arrest** on the table, and both **CPR** and the administration of **intralipid** fail to restore circulation, resulting in the patient's death.

## Question

Who should be **initially informed** following this critical incident?

A) Police
B) Clinical Director
C) General Medical Council (GMC)
D) Medical Director
E) Revalidation Officer

## Explanation

In cases of **serious medical errors** leading to patient harm or death, the **initial notification** should be made to the hospital's **Medical Director**. The Medical Director holds responsibility for overseeing the safety and governance of clinical care within the hospital. They will coordinate the subsequent investigation and reporting process and ensure that all relevant mandatory organizations, such as the **Care Quality Commission (CQC)**, are informed.

Once the **Medical Director** is informed, they will escalate the case as necessary to regulatory bodies, including the **General Medical Council (GMC)**, for further investigation of the clinicians involved. In cases of patient death, a **coroner** may also be involved, but the Medical Director handles these escalations.

It is not appropriate to contact the **Police** unless criminal negligence is suspected, and the **Revalidation Officer** is not involved in these matters.

## Advanced Surgical Talk

When medical errors occur, especially those resulting in severe consequences like death, it is crucial to follow a structured approach to incident reporting. The **Medical Director** is responsible for initiating a formal internal investigation to determine the root cause and manage the implications of the incident.

The process of reporting typically involves:

1. **Internal investigation** led by the Medical Director, involving the risk management and governance teams.

2. **External reporting** to regulatory agencies like the **Care Quality Commission (CQC)**, which ensures that care quality standards are maintained.

3. **Reporting to the GMC** if there are concerns about the clinical competence or actions of the healthcare professionals involved.

4. **Communication with the patient's family** under the **Duty of Candour**, ensuring transparency about the incident.

The **Medical Director** is the key figure in coordinating these steps and ensuring that all necessary parties are informed and appropriate actions are taken.

**Correct Answer: D) Medical Director**

### References

1. National Health Service (NHS). Being Open: Communicating patient safety incidents with patients and their carers. London: NHS; 2020.

2. General Medical Council (GMC). Raising and acting on concerns about patient safety. London: GMC; 2021.

## Case 42: Fluid Resuscitation in Sepsis

### Clinical Scenario

A 68-year-old man presents with septic shock and is being treated with intravenous fluids as part of the initial resuscitation. After receiving a substantial amount of crystalloids (e.g., normal saline or Hartmann's solution), his hemodynamic status has not improved. The team considers alternative fluids, including albumin, to further support his resuscitation efforts.

### Question

According to the **Surviving Sepsis Guidelines**, which of the following is the most appropriate next step in fluid management for a patient in septic shock who has not responded to substantial crystalloid resuscitation?

A) Continue with more crystalloid fluid
B) Use albumin as an adjunct to crystalloid
C) Use hydroxyethyl starch (HES)
D) Administer 5% dextrose solution
E) Use hypertonic saline

## Explanation

According to the **Surviving Sepsis Campaign Guidelines**, **albumin** is recommended as an adjunct to crystalloid fluids in patients with septic shock who have received substantial amounts of crystalloids but have not achieved adequate resuscitation. Albumin may be used to maintain plasma oncotic pressure and help achieve hemodynamic stabilization [1].

The use of **hydroxyethyl starches (HES)** is **not recommended** in patients with sepsis, as studies have shown that starches can be detrimental, leading to increased risks of **acute kidney injury (AKI)** and increased mortality [2]. For this reason, starches are avoided in fluid resuscitation for septic shock.

- **Crystalloids** remain the **first-line** fluids for resuscitation in septic shock, but when large volumes are insufficient to stabilize the patient, **albumin** can be added.

- **5% dextrose** and **hypertonic saline** are not appropriate for resuscitation in this context as they do not address the primary need for volume expansion and hemodynamic support.

## Advanced Surgical Talk

In septic shock, the **Surviving Sepsis Guidelines** recommend an initial bolus of **30 mL/kg of crystalloid** within the first 3 hours of recognition to achieve adequate perfusion and reverse the shock state. If this initial crystalloid resuscitation fails, **albumin** is suggested as an adjunct to help maintain intravascular volume [1]. Albumin, being a colloid, has a higher oncotic pressure compared to crystalloids, helping retain fluid within the vascular space and improve circulatory volume.

The use of **hydroxyethyl starches (HES)** in fluid resuscitation for sepsis has fallen out of favor due to evidence linking it to adverse outcomes, including increased rates of **acute kidney injury (AKI)** and **mortality** [2]. As a result, **starches are contraindicated** in the management of sepsis.

Fluid resuscitation should be continuously guided by frequent reassessment of the patient's hemodynamics and response to therapy. The goal is to restore tissue perfusion and prevent the progression of organ failure.

**Correct Answer: B) Use albumin as an adjunct to crystalloid**

**References**

1. Rhodes A, Evans LE, Alhazzani W, et al. Surviving Sepsis Campaign: International Guidelines for Management of Sepsis and Septic Shock: 2016. Crit Care Med. 2017;45(3):486-552.

2. Perner A, Haase N, Guttormsen AB, et al. Hydroxyethyl starch 130/0.42 versus Ringer's acetate in severe sepsis. N Engl J Med. 2012;367(2):124-34.

## Case 43: Timing of Antibiotic Administration in Suspected Sepsis

### Clinical Scenario

A 55-year-old woman presents to the emergency department with complaints of fever, shortness of breath, and confusion. Her blood pressure is 85/50 mmHg, heart rate is 120 beats per minute, and oxygen saturation is 89% on room air. On examination, she appears lethargic with a temperature of 39.1°C. Sepsis is suspected, and the team is preparing to start antibiotics.

### Question

What is the most appropriate timing for administering antibiotics in this patient, based on the **Surviving Sepsis Guidelines**?

A) Administer antimicrobials within 6 hours of presentation
B) Administer antimicrobials immediately, ideally within 1 hour of recognition
C) Wait for blood cultures to confirm infection before administering antimicrobials
D) Administer antimicrobials only if shock persists after initial fluid resuscitation
E) Administer antimicrobials within 3 hours if non-infectious causes are ruled out

### Explanation

This patient presents with **septic shock** as evidenced by her hypotension, tachycardia, and altered mental status. According to the **Surviving Sepsis Guidelines**, when **shock is present** or sepsis is deemed **definite or probable, antibiotics should be administered immediately, ideally within 1 hour of recognition** [1]. Early initiation of antimicrobial therapy is critical to improving outcomes in patients with septic shock, as delays in treatment are associated with increased mortality.

In cases where sepsis is **possible** but not definitive and the patient is **not in shock**, rapid assessment to rule out non-infectious causes is appropriate. However, when sepsis is probable or when shock is present, the priority is to start antimicrobials as quickly as possible [1].

**Advanced Surgical Talk**

The **Surviving Sepsis Guidelines** emphasize that early administration of antibiotics in sepsis and septic shock is crucial for reducing mortality. In patients presenting with **shock**, antibiotics should be started within **1 hour of recognition**. Rapid administration of antimicrobials helps to control the underlying infection and prevent further progression to multi-organ failure.

In cases where sepsis is suspected but the patient is not in shock, clinicians have up to **3 hours** to complete a **rapid assessment** of whether the cause of the acute illness is infectious or non-infectious [2]. If there is still concern for infection after this assessment, antibiotics should be started ( Table 3).

Delaying antimicrobial therapy while waiting for blood culture results is not advised, as blood cultures can take time and any delay in therapy can lead to worse outcomes. Instead, antibiotics should be started empirically based on the most likely source of infection, with subsequent adjustments made once culture results are available [1].

Correct Answer: B) Administer antimicrobials immediately, ideally within 1 hour of recognition

**References**


1.  Rhodes A, Evans LE, Alhazzani W, et al. Surviving Sepsis Campaign: International Guidelines for Management of Sepsis and Septic Shock: 2016. Crit Care Med. 2017;45(3):486-552.

2.  Levy MM, Evans LE, Rhodes A. The Surviving Sepsis Campaign Bundle: 2018 Update. Intensive Care Med. 2018;44(6):925-928.

*Table 3: Antibiotic timing in patients with sepsis*

| Sepsis Condition | Shock is Present | Shock is Absent |
| --- | --- | --- |
| **Sepsis is Definite or Probable** | Administer antimicrobials **immediately**, ideally within 1 hour of recognition | Rapid assessment of infectious vs non-infectious causes of illness |
| **Sepsis is Possible** | Administer antimicrobials **immediately**, ideally within 1 hour of recognition | Administer antimicrobials **within 3 hours** if concern for infection persists |

## Case 44: Vasopressor Use in Septic Shock

### Clinical Scenario

A 63-year-old man is admitted to the ICU with septic shock after presenting with fever, hypotension (blood pressure 80/45 mmHg), and tachycardia. Despite aggressive fluid resuscitation, his mean arterial pressure (MAP) remains low at 55 mmHg. The ICU team considers initiating vasopressors to maintain adequate perfusion and stabilize his blood pressure.

### Question

Which of the following is the most appropriate vasopressor strategy based on the **Surviving Sepsis Guidelines**?

A) Use dopamine as the first-line vasopressor
B) Use norepinephrine as the first-line vasopressor
C) Start vasopressors only after central access is secured
D) Add vasopressin as the first-line agent
E) Use epinephrine as the first-line vasopressor

### Explanation

In patients with septic shock who do not respond adequately to fluid resuscitation, vasopressors are required to maintain **mean arterial pressure (MAP)** and ensure adequate perfusion to vital organs. According to the **Surviving Sepsis Guidelines**, **norepinephrine** is recommended as the **first-line vasopressor** for managing septic shock [1]. The goal is to target a **MAP of 65 mmHg** to ensure sufficient organ perfusion.

- **Norepinephrine** is preferred over dopamine due to a lower risk of arrhythmias and better outcomes in septic shock.

- If **central venous access** is not yet available, **vasopressors can be initiated peripherally** in the short term but should be transitioned to central access as soon as possible.

- If the MAP is inadequate despite the use of norepinephrine, **vasopressin** can be added as a second-line agent.

- **Dobutamine** or **epinephrine** may be considered in cases of persistent cardiac dysfunction or hypoperfusion despite adequate volume resuscitation and vasopressor use [2].

### Advanced Surgical Talk

In the management of **septic shock**, restoring adequate perfusion pressure is critical to avoid organ failure. The **Surviving Sepsis Guidelines** recommend norepinephrine as the primary vasopressor due to its effectiveness in increasing blood pressure by vasoconstriction with a lower risk of side effects like arrhythmias compared to other agents such as dopamine [1].

**Vasopressor therapy** should begin as soon as possible when hypotension persists despite fluid resuscitation. The target **MAP of 65 mmHg** is recommended to maintain perfusion to the brain, heart, and kidneys. If peripheral vasopressors are used initially, they should be administered only for a short period and in a large vein (e.g., antecubital fossa) to minimize the risk of extravasation [2].

When a patient remains hypotensive despite moderate doses of norepinephrine, **vasopressin** is often added to help achieve the desired blood pressure. In cases of **cardiac dysfunction** with ongoing hypoperfusion despite adequate volume and vasopressor support, agents like **dobutamine** or **epinephrine** may be used ( Table 4).

Correct Answer: B) Use norepinephrine as the first-line vasopressor

### References

1. Rhodes A, Evans LE, Alhazzani W, et al. Surviving Sepsis Campaign: International Guidelines for Management of

Sepsis and Septic Shock: 2016. Crit Care Med. 2017;45(3):486-552.

   2. Levy MM, Evans LE, Rhodes A. The Surviving Sepsis Campaign Bundle: 2018 Update. Intensive Care Med. 2018;44(6):925-928

*Table 4: Vasoactive Agent Management in Septic Shock*

| Vasoactive Agent Recommendations | Details |
| --- | --- |
| **First-line vasopressor** | Use **norepinephrine** for patients with septic shock on vasopressors |
| **Target MAP (Mean Arterial Pressure)** | Target a **MAP of 65 mmHg** |
| **Central access not available** | Consider initiating vasopressors **peripherally** (for a short period of time) |
| **If MAP is inadequate with norepinephrine** | Consider adding **vasopressin** |
| **Invasive monitoring** | Consider invasive monitoring of **arterial blood pressure** |
| **Persistent cardiac dysfunction despite MAP** | Consider adding **dobutamine** or switching to **epinephrine** |

## Case 45: Rapid Sequence Induction

### Clinical Scenario

A 35-year-old man with a full stomach is brought to the emergency department for emergency surgery following a traumatic injury. Due to the risk of aspiration, the anaesthetist decides to perform **rapid sequence induction (RSI)**. The anaesthetic team prepares **thiopentone** for induction and discusses the considerations for RSI.

## Question

Which of the following statements is true regarding the use of **thiopentone** for rapid sequence induction (RSI)?

A) Thiopentone is suitable for both induction and maintenance of anaesthesia
B) Thiopentone has a slow onset and is not preferred for RSI
C) Thiopentone is frequently used for RSI due to its rapid onset but is unsuitable for maintenance
D) Thiopentone reduces the risk of aspiration during RSI
E) Thiopentone requires no additional considerations for airway protection during RSI

## Explanation

**Thiopentone** is a **barbiturate** with a **rapid onset** of action, making it ideal for **rapid sequence induction (RSI)**, where quick induction of anaesthesia is required to minimize the risk of aspiration. However, thiopentone is **not suitable for maintenance of anaesthesia** due to its pharmacokinetics, which lead to prolonged recovery times when used continuously.

During RSI, the rapid onset of thiopentone ensures that the patient is induced quickly, but other drugs are typically used for the **maintenance phase** of anaesthesia. Additionally, **cricoid pressure** is often applied during RSI to prevent regurgitation and aspiration by compressing the oesophagus.

It is important to note that while thiopentone is effective for **induction**, it does not reduce the risk of aspiration on its own. The risk of aspiration is managed by using cricoid pressure and quick securing of the airway.

### Advanced Surgical Talk

**Rapid sequence induction (RSI)** is a technique used in patients at high risk for aspiration, such as those with a full stomach or undergoing emergency surgery. The aim is to quickly induce anaesthesia and secure the airway with minimal delay. **Thiopentone** is commonly used for RSI due to its **rapid onset** (within seconds), ensuring that the patient is rendered unconscious quickly, allowing for prompt intubation.

However, thiopentone is **unsuitable for maintenance of anaesthesia** due to its pharmacological properties, which lead to slow elimination and potential accumulation in the body with prolonged use. Therefore, once induction is achieved, another anaesthetic agent, such as **propofol** or an inhalational agent, is typically used to maintain anaesthesia.

In RSI, there is always a risk of **aspiration** of gastric contents due to the rapid loss of consciousness and relaxation of the airway muscles. To mitigate this, **cricoid pressure** (Sellick's manoeuvre) is applied during intubation to compress the oesophagus and reduce the risk of regurgitation. This is a crucial step in RSI, especially in emergency scenarios [1].

**Correct Answer: C) Thiopentone is frequently used for RSI due to its rapid onset but is unsuitable for maintenance**

### References

1. Miller RD, Eriksson LI, Fleisher LA, et al. Miller's Anesthesia. 8th ed. Philadelphia: Elsevier; 2015.

2. Cook TM, Woodall N, Harper J, et al. Major complications of airway management in the UK: results of the 4th National Audit Project of the Royal College of Anaesthetists. Br J Anaesth. 2011;106(5):617-631.

## Case 46: Blood Types and Immunoglobulin Classes

### Clinical Scenario

A 30-year-old woman is undergoing preoperative evaluation, including blood typing, in preparation for elective surgery. The laboratory results reveal she has **blood type O**. The anaesthesiologist reviews her chart and notes that patients with different blood types may have different classes of **immunoglobulins (Ig)** related to their blood group antigens.

### Question

Which of the following statements correctly describes the immunoglobulin types associated with **blood type O** and **blood types A or B**?

A) Patients with blood type O produce IgM antibodies, while patients with blood types A or B produce IgG
B) Patients with blood type O produce IgG antibodies, while patients with blood types A or B produce IgM
C) All patients, regardless of blood type, produce IgM antibodies
D) Patients with blood type O produce IgA antibodies
E) Patients with blood type O and A produce IgG, while blood type B produces IgM

## Explanation

The type of immunoglobulin (Ig) produced in response to blood group antigens varies between **blood type O** and blood types **A or B**. Specifically:

- In **patients with blood type O**, the primary **Ig type is IgG**. Blood type O individuals have **anti-A** and **anti-B antibodies**, which are predominantly **IgG** antibodies [1].

- In **patients with blood types A or B**, the antibodies produced against the non-self blood group antigens (e.g., anti-B in type A individuals or anti-A in type B individuals) are primarily **IgM** antibodies [1][2].

This difference in the immunoglobulin class is significant for blood transfusion reactions and the risk of haemolytic reactions. **IgM** antibodies are more effective in activating the complement system and causing immediate haemolysis, while **IgG** antibodies can lead to a delayed haemolytic response [2].

### Advanced Surgical Talk

The distinction between **IgG** and **IgM** antibodies in relation to blood types is critical in transfusion medicine. **Blood type O** individuals produce **IgG antibodies** against **A** and **B antigens**, which is why they can only receive blood from other type O donors. These IgG antibodies are smaller and can cross the placenta, which is also important in **haemolytic disease of the newborn** [2].

On the other hand, individuals with **blood type A** or **blood type B** produce **IgM antibodies** against the opposite antigen. IgM antibodies are large and do not cross the placenta, but they are highly effective at activating the complement cascade, leading to immediate haemolysis in case of mismatched transfusion [1][2].

Understanding these immunoglobulin differences is essential when selecting compatible blood for transfusion and when managing conditions like **haemolytic reactions** or **blood type incompatibility** during pregnancy.

Correct Answer: B) Patients with blood type O produce IgG antibodies, while patients with blood types A or B produce IgM

### References

1. Daniels G. Human Blood Groups. 3rd ed. Wiley-Blackwell; 2013.

2.   Harmening DM. Modern Blood Banking & Transfusion Practices. 6th ed. Philadelphia: F.A. Davis; 2012

## Case 47: Blood Type and Rhogam Use in Pregnancy

### Clinical Scenario

A 32-year-old pregnant woman with **blood type A** and **Rh-negative** status is undergoing routine antenatal care. During a discussion with her obstetrician, she asks about the risk of her baby developing **haemolytic disease of the newborn (HDN)** due to blood type and Rh incompatibility. Her baby has been identified as having **blood type O** and is **Rh-positive**. The obstetrician explains that the risk of HDN is relatively low in her case.

### Question

Why is the risk of haemolytic disease of the newborn (HDN) considered **low** in this context, and what is the role of **Rhogam**?

A) The risk is high because IgM antibodies can cross the placenta and affect the baby
B) The risk is low because the maternal blood type produces IgM antibodies, which do not cross the placenta
C) The risk is high in the first pregnancy but low in subsequent pregnancies
D) The risk is higher because maternal blood type produces IgG antibodies that cross the placenta
E) Rhogam is given to prevent the production of maternal IgM antibodies

### Explanation

In this scenario, the **risk of haemolytic disease of the newborn (HDN)** due to **ABO incompatibility** is considered **low** because the maternal blood type produces **IgM antibodies**, which **do not cross the placenta**. This means that, although the mother's blood type is A and the baby's is O, the maternal anti-B antibodies are unlikely to harm the foetus. **IgM antibodies** are too large to cross the placenta and do not pose a threat to the foetus in this case [1].

However, the mother is **Rh-negative**, and the baby is **Rh-positive**, which presents a risk for **Rh sensitization**. If the mother becomes sensitized to the Rh-positive blood, she may produce **IgG antibodies** that could cross the placenta and cause haemolysis in future pregnancies. To prevent this, **Rhogam** (anti-D immunoglobulin) is administered at **28 weeks** and sometimes at

**34 weeks**, as well as within **72 hours** of delivery if the baby is confirmed to be Rh-positive. Rhogam prevents the mother from producing IgG antibodies that could attack Rh-positive foetal red blood cells in subsequent pregnancies [2].

Since the maternal antibodies in this case related to ABO incompatibility are **IgM**, and Rhogam prevents Rh sensitization, the risk of HDN in this pregnancy is low.

**Advanced Surgical Talk**

In **Rh incompatibility**, when a **Rh-negative mother** is carrying a **Rh-positive foetus**, there is a risk that maternal exposure to foetal red blood cells can lead to the development of **IgG antibodies** against the Rh antigen. These **IgG antibodies** can cross the placenta and attack the foetal red blood cells, leading to **haemolytic disease of the newborn (HDN)**. This is why **Rhogam** is administered to Rh-negative mothers carrying Rh-positive babies. Rhogam prevents the mother from becoming sensitized and producing these IgG antibodies [1].

In contrast, **ABO incompatibility** generally poses less risk in pregnancy because the maternal antibodies (anti-A or anti-B) are primarily **IgM**, which do not cross the placenta. Even though the mother has **blood type A** and the baby has **blood type O**, the risk of significant haemolysis is low because IgM antibodies are not transferred to the foetus. The focus in this case is on **Rh incompatibility**, which can lead to **IgG** formation and affect future pregnancies if Rhogam is not given [2].

Correct Answer: B) The risk is low because the maternal blood type produces IgM antibodies, which do not cross the placenta

**References**


1.  Daniels G. Human Blood Groups. 3rd ed. Wiley-Blackwell; 2013.

2.  Harmening DM. Modern Blood Banking & Transfusion Practices. 6th ed. Philadelphia: F.A. Davis; 2012

# Case 48: qSOFA Score and Sepsis Outcome Prediction

## Clinical Scenario

A 65-year-old woman presents to the emergency department with confusion, hypotension (blood pressure 85/50 mmHg), and a respiratory rate of 30 breaths per minute. Her pulse is 120 beats per minute, and she has a history of diabetes and chronic kidney disease. The clinical team suspects she might have sepsis, and they calculate her **qSOFA score** as part of her assessment.

## Question

What is the significance of this patient's **qSOFA score of 3**, and how should it be interpreted in the context of sepsis?

A) qSOFA is used to diagnose sepsis
B) A qSOFA score of 3 indicates a higher risk of poor outcomes and the need to consider sepsis
C) A qSOFA score of 3 indicates the need for immediate antibiotic administration
D) qSOFA score is only relevant in ICU settings
E) qSOFA is only used in conjunction with blood cultures

## Explanation

**qSOFA** (quick Sequential Organ Failure Assessment) is a scoring system used to identify patients at risk of poor outcomes from sepsis. It is not used to **diagnose sepsis** itself, but rather to identify patients who may be at risk for **worse outcomes** and should prompt clinicians to consider sepsis as a possible cause. The **qSOFA score** is calculated based on the following criteria:

- **Respiratory rate ≥22 breaths/min**

- **Altered mental status**

- **Systolic blood pressure ≤100 mmHg**

Each criterion scores **1 point**, and a score of **2 or more** indicates an increased risk of poor outcomes. In this case, the patient has a qSOFA score of **3** (due to her altered mental status, hypotension, and tachypnoea), which suggests a **higher risk of mortality** or adverse outcomes. This score should prompt urgent evaluation and management, including considering sepsis as a potential cause of her condition [1].

**qSOFA is not used to diagnose sepsis**, but it helps clinicians identify patients who may have sepsis and require further workup and intervention. The patient's qSOFA score suggests that she is at high risk for poor outcomes and should be treated urgently [2].

**Advanced Surgical Talk**

The **qSOFA score** was developed as a simple bedside tool to quickly identify patients who are at risk of poor outcomes due to sepsis. It does not replace the full **SOFA (Sequential Organ Failure Assessment)** score, which is more detailed and used in the **ICU** setting to assess the degree of organ dysfunction in septic patients. However, **qSOFA** is useful in emergency departments and wards to quickly assess patients.

In this case, the patient's **qSOFA score of 3** indicates that she is at high risk for deterioration and death due to sepsis, and it should prompt immediate management, including **fluid resuscitation**, **antibiotics**, and close monitoring. It is important to remember that **qSOFA is not a diagnostic tool for sepsis**, but rather a **predictor of worse outcomes** [1][3].

Correct Answer: B) A qSOFA score of 3 indicates a higher risk of poor outcomes and the need to consider sepsis

**References**


1.  Seymour CW, Liu VX, Iwashyna TJ, et al. Assessment of Clinical Criteria for Sepsis: For the Third International Consensus Definitions for Sepsis and Septic Shock (Sepsis-3). JAMA. 2016;315(8):762-774.

2.  Singer M, Deutschman CS, Seymour CW, et al. The Third International Consensus Definitions for Sepsis and Septic Shock (Sepsis-3). JAMA. 2016;315(8):801-810.

3.  Rhodes A, Evans LE, Alhazzani W, et al. Surviving Sepsis Campaign: International Guidelines for Management of Sepsis and Septic Shock: 2016. Crit Care Med. 2017;45(3):486-552.


## qSOFA and SOFA

**qSOFA** (quick Sequential Organ Failure Assessment) and **SOFA** (Sequential Organ Failure Assessment) differ in several important ways, primarily in their purpose, complexity, and use cases ( Table 5).

**1. Purpose:**

- **qSOFA:**
  - o It is a quick bedside tool designed to identify patients who are at risk of having poor outcomes from sepsis. It does **not** diagnose sepsis but serves as a **screening tool** to trigger further investigation and management if sepsis is suspected.
  - o qSOFA is particularly useful in **non-ICU settings** (such as emergency departments or hospital wards) where time is critical, and a rapid assessment of sepsis risk is needed.

- **SOFA:**
  - o The full SOFA score is a more **comprehensive tool** used primarily in **ICU settings**. It helps to evaluate the extent of **organ dysfunction** in patients with suspected sepsis or other critical illnesses.
  - o SOFA is also used to **track the progression** of organ failure over time, making it valuable for **monitoring** critically ill patients in intensive care.

**2. Components:**

- **qSOFA:**
  - o **qSOFA** is much simpler and includes **3 criteria**, each worth 1 point:
    1. **Respiratory rate ≥ 22 breaths per minute**
    2. **Systolic blood pressure ≤ 100 mmHg**
    3. **Altered mental status** (Glasgow Coma Scale < 15)

A score of **2 or more** suggests a higher risk of poor outcomes and should prompt clinicians to consider sepsis and take action.

- **SOFA:**
  - o The full **SOFA score** evaluates **6 organ systems** and assigns points based on the level of dysfunction in each:
    1. **Respiratory system** ($PaO_2/FiO_2$ ratio)
    2. **Coagulation** (platelet count)

3. **Liver function** (bilirubin level)

4. **Cardiovascular function** (mean arterial pressure and use of vasopressors)

5. **Central nervous system** (Glasgow Coma Scale score)

6. **Renal function** (creatinine level or urine output)

The total SOFA score can range from **0 to 24**, with higher scores indicating greater organ dysfunction and a higher risk of mortality.

## 3. Complexity:

- **qSOFA:**
  - It is **simple and quick** to calculate without the need for laboratory results or advanced equipment. It is intended to be used at the **bedside** in non-ICU settings.

- **SOFA:**
  - SOFA requires **lab tests** and measurements of various organ systems, making it more **complex** and suitable for use in **ICU settings**, where detailed tracking of organ function over time is essential.

## 4. Use Cases:

- **qSOFA:**
  - Used in **non-ICU** settings (e.g., emergency departments, hospital wards) to **quickly assess** patients at risk for poor outcomes from sepsis. It is designed as a **screening tool** for clinicians to identify patients who might need further investigation for sepsis.

- **SOFA:**
  - Primarily used in **ICU settings** to assess the **severity of organ dysfunction** in critically ill patients, including those with sepsis. It is used to **track the progression** of a patient's illness and guide **treatment decisions**.

## *Table 5: qSOFA and SOFA differences*

| Feature | qSOFA | SOFA |
|---|---|---|
| **Purpose** | Identifies patients at risk for poor outcomes in sepsis (screening tool) | Assesses and tracks organ dysfunction in critically ill patients |
| **Components** | 3 criteria: altered mental status, respiratory rate, blood pressure | 6 organ systems: respiratory, coagulation, liver, cardiovascular, CNS, renal |
| **Setting** | Non-ICU settings (e.g., ED, hospital wards) | ICU settings |
| **Scoring** | Simple, quick bedside tool (score 0–3) | Comprehensive, requires lab data (score 0–24) |
| **Use** | Rapid screening for potential sepsis | Monitoring severity and progression of organ failure |

**Conclusion:**

- **qSOFA** is a quick tool to identify patients who may be at risk for sepsis and poor outcomes in **non-ICU settings**. It does not diagnose sepsis but helps identify patients who need urgent care.

- **SOFA** is a more detailed scoring system used in **ICU settings** to evaluate the extent of **organ failure** and guide treatment decisions for critically ill patients, including those with sepsis.

Both scores serve different purposes in managing patients with sepsis, but they are part of the continuum of care in identifying and treating patients at risk of sepsis and organ dysfunction.

## Clinical Scenario

A 62-year-old man presents for preoperative assessment before elective surgery. He is a current smoker but otherwise has no major health issues. However, he had a **myocardial infarction (MI)** two months ago. The anaesthesiology team is determining his **ASA classification** (American Society of Anaesthesiologists Physical Status Classification) based on his medical history.

## Question

Based on the patient's recent myocardial infarction and smoking history, what is his **ASA classification**?

A) ASA I
B) ASA II
C) ASA III
D) ASA IV
E) ASA V

## Explanation

The **ASA classification system** is used to assess a patient's preoperative health and predict perioperative risk. It ranges from **ASA I (normal healthy patient) to ASA V (moribund patient not expected to survive without the operation)**. The presence of **recent myocardial infarction (MI)** and smoking status affects the patient's ASA score:

- **ASA II**: A patient with **mild systemic disease** that does not limit activity (e.g., controlled hypertension, smoking, or mild obesity).

- **ASA III**: A patient with **severe systemic disease** that limits activity but is not incapacitating (e.g., poorly controlled diabetes or hypertension, a history of MI more than 3 months ago).

- **ASA IV**: A patient with **severe systemic disease that is a constant threat to life** (e.g., recent MI within the last 3 months, ongoing cardiac ischemia, or severe valvular dysfunction).

Since this patient had a **myocardial infarction less than 3 months ago**, he is placed in the **ASA IV** category, as recent MI poses a **significant risk of perioperative complications**.

Without the recent MI, his smoking habit would have placed him in **ASA II**.

**Advanced Surgical Talk**

The **ASA classification** is a valuable tool in preoperative risk stratification. Patients with **recent myocardial infarction (MI)** are at high risk for **perioperative complications**, including reinfarction, heart failure, and death. The ASA IV classification reflects the seriousness of a recent MI and indicates that surgery in such patients should be carefully evaluated and may need to be delayed if possible, to reduce risk.

Smoking also contributes to systemic disease, but without the MI, this patient's smoking status alone would place him in the **ASA II** category. Smokers are at increased risk of respiratory and cardiovascular complications during and after surgery, but this is generally considered a **mild systemic disease** in the context of ASA classification [1].

Patients with **recent MI** require careful monitoring and potentially **optimization** of their cardiovascular status before undergoing elective surgery. In most cases, elective surgery should be postponed until **at least 3–6 months** after the MI to reduce the risk of complications [2].

**Correct Answer: D) ASA IV**

**References**


1.  Doyle DJ, Garmon EH. American Society of Anesthesiologists Classification (ASA Class). StatPearls. 2023.

2.  Fleisher LA, Fleischmann KE, Auerbach AD, et al. 2014 ACC/AHA Guideline on Perioperative Cardiovascular Evaluation and Management of Patients Undergoing Noncardiac Surgery. J Am Coll Cardiol. 2014;64(22).


## Case 50: Buffering Solutions to Reduce Injection Discomfort

**Clinical Scenario**

A 45-year-old woman presents for minor surgery under local anaesthesia. During the preoperative discussion, she mentions previous experiences of discomfort with local anaesthetic injections. The surgical team discusses ways to reduce the discomfort associated with local anaesthetic administration and considers using **buffering solutions**.

## Question

What is the benefit of using **buffering solutions** in local anaesthetic injections, and what does evidence suggest about their effectiveness?

A) Buffering solutions decrease the effectiveness of local anaesthetics
B) Buffering solutions increase the onset time of local anaesthetics
C) Buffering solutions reduce the discomfort associated with local anaesthetic injections
D) Buffering solutions increase the risk of systemic toxicity
E) Buffering solutions should only be used for major surgeries

## Explanation

**Buffering solutions**, such as **sodium bicarbonate**, are often added to local anaesthetics to **reduce the acidity** of the solution. This reduction in acidity helps minimize the **pain and discomfort** experienced by patients during injection. The addition of buffering solutions is especially beneficial when using local anaesthetics that are more acidic, such as **lidocaine**.

There is **strong evidence**, including a **Cochrane review**, supporting the use of buffering agents in local anaesthetics to reduce the discomfort associated with their administration. The Cochrane review suggests that adding buffering agents like sodium bicarbonate can significantly **decrease the pain** of injection without compromising the effectiveness or safety of the anaesthetic [1].

- **Buffering** does not decrease the effectiveness of local anaesthetics, and in fact, may **improve the onset time** by increasing the amount of active (non-ionized) form of the anaesthetic.

- The use of buffering agents is generally safe and does not increase the risk of systemic toxicity.

- Buffering solutions can be used in various types of surgeries, including minor procedures, to improve patient comfort.

## Advanced Surgical Talk

**Buffering local anaesthetic solutions** is a simple and effective method to improve patient comfort during procedures requiring local anaesthesia. Local anaesthetics like **lidocaine** are typically formulated at a low pH to increase their stability, but this acidity can cause a burning sensation when injected. By adding **sodium bicarbonate** or another buffering solution, the pH is raised, making the injection more comfortable for the patient.

The **Cochrane review** on this topic confirmed that buffering local anaesthetics leads to a **significant reduction in pain** during injection without affecting the anaesthetic's efficacy or safety profile [1]. Buffering is especially useful in procedures where multiple local anaesthetic injections are required, such as dental procedures or minor surgical interventions.

This technique is recommended for routine use in **minor surgeries** or any setting where local anaesthetic injections are likely to cause discomfort. Buffering also may **improve the onset time** of the anaesthetic, as the higher pH increases the amount of non-ionized anaesthetic, which more readily crosses nerve membranes to exert its effect.

Correct Answer: C) Buffering solutions reduce the discomfort associated with local anaesthetic injections

### References

1.  Cochrane Database of Systematic Reviews. Buffered versus unbuffered local anaesthetic for pain reduction during injection. Cochrane Library. 2021

---

## Case 51: ASA Classification

### Clinical Scenario

A 52-year-old man presents for preoperative evaluation before elective hernia repair surgery. He has a history of well-controlled hypertension and is otherwise healthy. During the assessment, he mentions that although he is able to perform all necessary self-care activities, he has been **unable to carry out his work duties** for the past few months. The anaesthesiologist is determining his **ASA classification** (American Society of Anaesthesiologists Physical Status Classification) based on his medical status and ability to function.

### Question

What is the most appropriate **ASA classification** for this patient?

A) ASA I
B) ASA II

C) ASA III
D) ASA IV
E) ASA V

**Explanation**

The **ASA classification system** is used to assess a patient's overall health status before surgery, categorizing patients from **ASA I** (healthy) to **ASA V** (moribund). Patients with mild systemic disease that does not limit daily activity are typically placed in the **ASA II** category. This classification includes patients with well-controlled medical conditions (e.g., hypertension, diabetes) that do not significantly impact their ability to perform daily tasks.

- In this case, the patient's **hypertension** is well-controlled, which qualifies as a **mild systemic disease**.

- Although the patient states that he is **unable to carry out work duties**, this is not due to a severe medical condition but may be related to personal or lifestyle choices. As long as his condition does not limit essential activities of daily living (e.g., self-care), he would still fall into the **ASA II** category.

Patients classified as **ASA III** or higher typically have more severe systemic disease that significantly limits daily activities. Since this patient can still perform self-care, he remains in the **ASA II** category.

**Advanced Surgical Talk**

The **ASA classification** system is used widely in preoperative assessments to estimate the **risk of perioperative complications** based on a patient's underlying health. In this case, the patient is classified as **ASA II** because his medical condition (well-controlled hypertension) is mild and does not limit his ability to perform **self-care** activities. Even though he states he cannot carry out work duties, this is not necessarily reflective of a higher ASA classification, unless it is directly due to a systemic disease that impacts his functional capacity.

In **ASA II** patients, perioperative risk is generally low, but the presence of mild systemic disease means the patient may require closer monitoring during surgery compared to **ASA I** patients, who are completely healthy.

It is also important to consider how patients' perceptions of their own abilities and lifestyle factors might influence their reported limitations. In cases where the limitations are not directly related to systemic disease, these factors should not elevate the patient's ASA classification unnecessarily [1][2].

**Correct Answer: B) ASA II**

## References


1. Doyle DJ, Garmon EH. American Society of Anesthesiologists Classification (ASA Class). StatPearls. 2023.

2. American Society of Anesthesiologists. ASA Physical Status Classification System. 2020. Available at: https://www.asahq.org.


---

## Case 52: Performance Status Assessment

### Clinical Scenario

A 60-year-old man, previously healthy, comes to the clinic with complaints of abdominal pain, fever, and changes in bowel habits. He is diagnosed with **diverticulitis** and has been prescribed antibiotics. During the consultation, he mentions that while he is able to perform all activities of **self-care**, he has been **unable to carry out his work duties** since the onset of his symptoms.

### Question

What is the most appropriate **performance status (PS)** classification for this patient based on his current condition?

A) PS 0
B) PS 1
C) PS 2
D) PS 3
E) PS 5

### Explanation

Performance status (PS) is a measure of a patient's overall physical functioning and ability to perform daily activities.

### Full ECOG Performance Status Scale:

- **PS 0**: Fully active, able to carry on all pre-disease activities without restriction.

- **PS 1**: Restricted in physically strenuous activity but able to carry out light work or daily activities.

- **PS 2**: Able to perform self-care, but unable to carry out work duties. Ambulatory for more than 50% of the time.

- **PS 3**: Capable of limited self-care, confined to a bed or chair for more than 50% of the day.

- **PS 4**: Completely disabled, unable to perform any self-care, totally confined to bed or chair.

- **PS 5**: Dead.

In this case, the patient is able to perform **self-care** but cannot carry out his **work duties** due to his diverticulitis symptoms. Therefore, his performance status is classified as **PS 2**, indicating moderate impairment.

## Advanced Surgical Talk

The **performance status (PS)** classification is an important tool used to assess a patient's ability to perform daily activities and their overall physical function. This can guide decision-making in both acute and chronic medical conditions, as it helps to determine a patient's **treatment tolerance** and prognosis. In this case, the patient's **PS 2** status suggests he can manage basic activities like eating, bathing, and dressing, but his condition prevents him from performing work-related tasks, which may involve more strenuous activity.

**PS 2** is often seen in patients with acute conditions like **diverticulitis**, where symptoms temporarily impair their ability to work but do not severely limit their daily living activities. **Self-care** is still maintained, and recovery can lead to an improvement in performance status with proper treatment [1][2].

Correct Answer: C) PS 2

## References


1. Oken MM, Creech RH, Tormey DC, et al. Toxicity and response criteria of the Eastern Cooperative Oncology Group. Am J Clin Oncol. 1982;5(6):649-55.

2. Karnofsky DA, Burchenal JH. The clinical evaluation of chemotherapeutic agents in cancer. In: Evaluation of Chemotherapeutic Agents. New York: Columbia Univ Press; 1949.

## Clinical Scenario

A 58-year-old woman undergoes a midline laparotomy for bowel resection. The surgical team is discussing the best suture material and technique for closing the abdominal wall to reduce the risk of incisional hernias. Traditionally, **1 loop PDS** (polydiaxonone) has been used for closure, but the team is considering recent evidence from the **STITCH trial**.

## Question

Which suture material and technique is recommended based on the **STITCH trial** to reduce the risk of incisional hernia formation?

A) 1 loop PDS with larger bites
B) 2/0 PDS with smaller bites
C) Polyglactin 910 (Vicryl) with larger bites
D) Polyglyconate (Maxon) with smaller bites
E) 1 loop Vicryl with large bites

## Explanation

**Polydiaxonone (PDS)** is a common choice for closing abdominal incisions due to its long-lasting absorbable properties. Traditionally, **1 loop PDS** was used, with surgeons often taking larger bites of the abdominal wall fascia to secure the closure. However, the **STITCH trial** demonstrated that using **smaller bites** with a finer suture, such as **2/0 PDS**, leads to a **significant reduction in incisional hernia rates** [1].

This technique focuses on placing sutures closer together and taking smaller bites of the tissue to achieve a more evenly distributed tension across the wound, leading to better healing and fewer incisional hernias.

- **Polyglactin 910 (Vicryl)** is a faster-absorbing suture used in many procedures, but it is not the preferred material for long-term abdominal wall closure due to its shorter absorption time.

- **Polyglyconate (Maxon)** is another absorbable suture, but it was not evaluated in the context of the **STITCH trial**.

The evidence suggests that **2/0 PDS** with **smaller bites** is the most effective technique for reducing the risk of incisional hernias in midline laparotomy closures.

**Advanced Surgical Talk**

The **STITCH trial** was a landmark study that compared different techniques and materials for closing abdominal wall incisions to reduce the incidence of **incisional hernias**. The trial showed that using **smaller bites** (5-8 mm from the wound edge) and **closer suture intervals** with **2/0 PDS** significantly lowered the rate of incisional hernia formation compared to traditional techniques that used larger bites.

This technique promotes better tissue healing by distributing tension more evenly across the wound and reducing the risk of suture pull-through and dehiscence. **Polydiaxonone (PDS)** is preferred for this type of closure due to its **long absorption profile**, providing prolonged wound support during the critical healing period [1][2].

Using smaller bites has since become a recommended practice, particularly in patients at high risk of hernia formation after abdominal surgery.

**Correct Answer: B) 2/0 PDS with smaller bites**

**References**


1. Deerenberg EB, Harlaar JJ, Steyerberg EW, et al. Small bites versus large bites for closure of abdominal midline incisions (STITCH trial): a double-blind, multicentre, randomised controlled trial. Lancet. 2015;386(10000):1254-1260.

2. Diener MK, Voss S, Jensen K, et al. Elective midline laparotomy closure: the INLINE systematic review and meta-analysis. Ann Surg. 2010;251(5):843-856.


## Case 54: Sensitivity Calculation

**Clinical Scenario**

A new diagnostic test is being evaluated for its ability to detect a particular disease. The test was performed on 50 patients, and the results are as follows:

- **True Positives (TP):** 20
- **False Negatives (FN):** 5
- **True Negatives (TN):** 25

The clinical team is asked to calculate the **sensitivity** of the test.

## Question

What is the **sensitivity** of the diagnostic test based on the given data?

A) 66%
B) 71%
C) 80%
D) 85%
E) 90%

## Explanation

**Sensitivity** is a measure of a diagnostic test's ability to correctly identify patients who have the disease (i.e., the proportion of **true positives** among those who actually have the disease). Sensitivity is calculated using the following formula:

Sensitivity=True Positives (TP)/True Positives (TP)+False Negatives (FN)

In this case:

- **True Positives (TP)** = 20

- **False Negatives (FN)** = 5

Sensitivity=20/20+5=0.80

So, the **sensitivity** of the test is **80%**.

## Advanced Surgical Talk

**Sensitivity** is one of the key parameters used to evaluate the performance of diagnostic tests. A highly sensitive test is useful for **screening**, as it correctly identifies most patients with the disease, minimizing the number of **false negatives**. In this case, the test correctly identifies **80%** of the true positive cases, which means that 20% of the actual cases are missed (false negatives).

The **specificity** of a test, which measures the proportion of **true negatives**, would also be important in evaluating this test, but it is not calculated in this example. Sensitivity and specificity are typically used together to fully understand the diagnostic accuracy of a test [1].

**Correct Answer: C) 80%**

### References

1. Parikh R, Mathai A, Parikh S, Chandra Sekhar G, Thomas R. Understanding and using sensitivity, specificity, and predictive values. Indian J Ophthalmol. 2008;56(1):45-50.

## Case 55: Specificity Calculation

### Clinical Scenario

A diagnostic test is being evaluated for its ability to correctly identify patients **without the disease**. The following data is available from 50 patients who underwent the test:

- **True Positives (TP)**: 20
- **False Negatives (FN)**: 5
- **True Negatives (TN)**: 25
- **False Positives (FP)**: 0

The clinical team is asked to calculate the **specificity** of the test.

### Question

What is the **specificity** of the diagnostic test based on the given data?

A) 80%
B) 85%
C) 90%
D) 95%
E) 100%

### Explanation

**Specificity** measures a test's ability to correctly identify those **without the disease** (i.e., the proportion of **true negatives** among all individuals who do not have the disease). The formula for calculating specificity is:

Specificity=True Negatives (TN)/True Negatives (TN)+False Positives

In this case:

- **True Negatives (TN)** = 25
- **False Positives (FP)** = 0

Specificity=25/25+0=1.0=100%

Since there are no false positives in this scenario, the test perfectly identifies all true negatives, meaning the **specificity is 100%**.

### Advanced Surgical Talk

**Specificity** is a critical measure in the evaluation of a diagnostic test, particularly in situations where it is important to **rule out disease** in patients who do not have it. A test with **high specificity** produces very few **false positives**, ensuring that healthy individuals are not incorrectly diagnosed with the disease.

In this case, the test's specificity is **100%**, meaning that all patients who do not have the disease were correctly identified as negative. In clinical practice, high specificity is especially valuable in confirming diagnoses, as it minimizes the risk of false positive results leading to unnecessary treatments [1].

**Correct Answer: E) 100%**

### References

1. Parikh R, Mathai A, Parikh S, Chandra Sekhar G, Thomas R. Understanding and using sensitivity, specificity, and predictive values. Indian J Ophthalmol. 2008;56(1):45-50.

## Case 56: Negative Predictive Value Calculation

### Clinical Scenario

A diagnostic test is being evaluated for its ability to predict **true negatives**, ensuring that patients who test negative truly do not have the disease. The following data is available from 50 patients who underwent the test:

- **True Positives (TP)**: 20
- **False Negatives (FN)**: 5
- **True Negatives (TN)**: 25
- **False Positives (FP)**: 0

The clinical team is asked to calculate the **negative predictive value (NPV)** of the test.

## Question

What is the **negative predictive value (NPV)** of the diagnostic test based on the given data?

A) 66%
B) 75%
C) 80%
D) 90%
E) 100%

## Explanation

The **negative predictive value (NPV)** indicates the probability that a patient with a negative test result truly does not have the disease. It is calculated using the following formula:

NPV=True Negatives (TN)/True Negatives (TN)+False Negatives ( FN)

In this case:

- **True Negatives (TN)** = 25

- **False Negatives (FN)** = 5

NPV=25/25+5=0.833=83.3%

So, the **negative predictive value** of the test is **83.3%**, meaning that 83.3% of the patients who test negative truly do not have the disease.

## Advanced Surgical Talk

**Negative predictive value (NPV)** is an important metric in clinical practice because it helps determine the likelihood that a **negative test result** truly indicates the absence of disease. In this case, the NPV of **83.3%** suggests that the test is quite reliable in ruling out disease in patients who test negative, though some cases (16.7%) may still be missed due to false negatives.

NPV depends not only on the characteristics of the test (e.g., sensitivity and specificity) but also on the **prevalence** of the disease in the population being tested. In a population with **low disease prevalence**, NPV tends to be higher, because more people do not have the disease, making it more likely that a negative result is accurate [1].

**Correct Answer: C) 80%**(approximately)


## References

1.   Parikh R, Mathai A, Parikh S, Chandra Sekhar G, Thomas R. Understanding and using sensitivity, specificity, and predictive values. Indian J Ophthalmol. 2008;56(1):45-50.

## Case 57: False Positive Rate Calculation

### Clinical Scenario

A diagnostic test is being evaluated for its **false positive rate**. The test results for 50 patients are as follows:

- **True Positives (TP)**: 20
- **False Negatives (FN)**: 5
- **True Negatives (TN)**: 25
- **False Positives (FP)**: 0

The clinical team is asked to calculate the **false positive rate** of the test.

### Question

What is the **false positive rate** of the diagnostic test based on the given data?

A) 0%
B) 5%
C) 10%
D) 20%
E) 50%

### Explanation

The **false positive rate** (FPR) is the probability that a patient without the disease will test **positive**. It is calculated using the following formula:

False Positive Rate (FPR)=False Positives (FP)/False Positives (FP)+True Negatives (TN)

In this case:

- **False Positives (FP)** = 0
- **True Negatives (TN)** = 25

FPR=0/0+25=025=0%

Since there were no false positives in this scenario, the **false positive rate is 0%**.

## Advanced Surgical Talk

The **false positive rate (FPR)** is an important metric when evaluating the accuracy of diagnostic tests, particularly when testing healthy individuals. A **low FPR** means that the test is unlikely to **incorrectly identify** healthy individuals as having the disease. In this case, because there were **no false positives**, the FPR is **0%**, which indicates that the test has performed well in accurately identifying individuals who do not have the disease.

This metric is closely related to **specificity**, which measures the test's ability to correctly identify those without the disease. A **high specificity** results in a **low false positive rate** [1].

**Correct Answer: A) 0%**

## References

1. Parikh R, Mathai A, Parikh S, Chandra Sekhar G, Thomas R. Understanding and using sensitivity, specificity, and predictive values. Indian J Ophthalmol. 2008;56(1):45-50.

## Case 58: Mechanism of Action of Antithrombin III

### Clinical Scenario

A 50-year-old man is started on **anticoagulant therapy** following a diagnosis of deep vein thrombosis (DVT). The chosen anticoagulant works by binding to **antithrombin III** and enhancing its ability to inactivate **thrombin**. The patient asks how the medication works and its role in preventing clot formation.

### Question

What is the **mechanism of action** of the anticoagulant described in this scenario?

A) Direct thrombin inhibitor
B) Factor Xa inhibitor
C) Antithrombin III activator
D) Vitamin K antagonist
E) Fibrinolytic agent

### Explanation

The anticoagulant described in this case works by binding to **antithrombin III**, a natural protein in the body that inhibits **thrombin** and **factor Xa**, key components in the clotting cascade. This type of anticoagulant is known as an **antithrombin III activator** [1].

**Heparin** is the most common example of an antithrombin III activator. By binding to antithrombin III, heparin increases its inhibitory activity, which leads to the **inactivation of thrombin** and **factor Xa**, ultimately preventing clot formation [2].

Other anticoagulants that work via **direct thrombin inhibition** or **factor Xa inhibition** have different mechanisms and do not rely on antithrombin III.

## Advanced Surgical Talk

**Antithrombin III** is a natural inhibitor of clot formation that primarily inactivates **thrombin (factor IIa)** and **factor Xa**. **Heparin**, both unfractionated and low-molecular-weight forms (e.g., enoxaparin), binds to and enhances the activity of **antithrombin III**, leading to rapid inactivation of these clotting factors [1].

This mechanism makes antithrombin III activators very effective in the acute management of conditions such as **deep vein thrombosis (DVT)**, **pulmonary embolism**, and **acute coronary syndromes**. These agents act rapidly and are often used in settings where immediate anticoagulation is needed, such as perioperatively or in hospitalized patients [2].

Correct Answer: C) Antithrombin III activator

## References


1. Weitz JI, Eikelboom JW, Samama MM. New antithrombotic drugs: Antithrombotic therapy and prevention of thrombosis. Chest. 2012;141(2 Suppl).

2. Hirsh J, Raschke R. Heparin and low-molecular-weight heparin: the Seventh ACCP Conference on Antithrombotic and Thrombolytic Therapy. Chest. 2004;126(3 Suppl):188S-203S.

## Clinical Scenario

A 68-year-old man undergoes elective bowel surgery. Postoperatively, he develops significant complications, including organ failure that requires admission to the intensive care unit (ICU). Despite aggressive treatment, the patient unfortunately passes away.

## Question

How would this complication be classified according to the **Clavien-Dindo classification system**?

A) Clavien-Dindo 1
B) Clavien-Dindo 2
C) Clavien-Dindo 3
D) Clavien-Dindo 4
E) Clavien-Dindo 5

## Explanation

The **Clavien-Dindo classification** is a widely used system for grading surgical complications based on their severity. The classification ranges from **Grade 1 (minor complications)** to **Grade 5 (death)**:

- **Clavien-Dindo 1**: Any deviation from the normal postoperative course without the need for pharmacological treatment or surgical, endoscopic, or radiological interventions.

- **Clavien-Dindo 2**: Complications requiring pharmacological treatment (e.g., antibiotics, blood transfusions).

- **Clavien-Dindo 3**: Complications requiring surgical, endoscopic, or radiological intervention.

- **Clavien-Dindo 4**: Life-threatening complications requiring intensive care management (e.g., organ failure).

- **Clavien-Dindo 5**: Death of the patient.

In this scenario, the patient developed complications that resulted in **death**, which is classified as a **Clavien-Dindo 5** complication, the most severe category in the system [1].

**Advanced Surgical Talk**

The **Clavien-Dindo classification system** is an essential tool in assessing and reporting postoperative complications. It allows for standardized reporting of complications based on their severity and the interventions required to manage them. This system is valuable for improving quality control in surgery and for comparing outcomes across different procedures and institutions.

In this case, since the patient unfortunately died as a result of postoperative complications, the event is classified as a **Clavien-Dindo 5** complication. Other grades in the system would apply if the patient had survived but required ICU admission (Clavien-Dindo 4) or a less intensive intervention (Clavien-Dindo 3) [1][2].

**Correct Answer: E) Clavien-Dindo 5**

## References

1. Dindo D, Demartines N, Clavien PA. Classification of surgical complications: a new proposal with evaluation in a cohort of 6336 patients and results of a survey. Ann Surg. 2004;240(2):205-213.

2. Clavien PA, Barkun J, de Oliveira ML, et al. The Clavien-Dindo classification of surgical complications: five-year experience. Ann Surg. 2009;250(2):187-196.

---

## Case 60: Genetic Modelling in Research

### Clinical Scenario

A team of researchers is conducting a study on genetic mutations and their potential impact on disease development. Instead of using animal models or laboratory experiments, they decide to perform their study using **computer-based simulations** to model gene interactions and predict outcomes.

### Question

What is the term used to describe the method of using **computer-based simulations** in genetic research?

A) In vivo
B) In vitro
C) In situ
D) In silico
E) Ex vivo

## Explanation

The term **in silico** refers to the use of **computer-based simulations** in scientific research, particularly for modelling biological processes, such as genetic interactions and disease pathways. **In silico** methods are commonly used in **genetic modelling studies** to predict the effects of mutations, explore gene interactions, and simulate biological processes without needing to perform experiments on living organisms or in the lab [1].

- **In vivo** refers to experiments conducted within a living organism.

- **In vitro** refers to experiments performed outside of a living organism, usually in a controlled laboratory environment (e.g., petri dishes or test tubes).

- **In situ** refers to observations or experiments conducted in the original location or natural environment of the subject.

- **Ex vivo** refers to experiments conducted on tissues or cells taken from an organism, but outside the body.

In this case, **in silico** methods are the correct term for the approach the researchers are using.

## Advanced Surgical Talk

**In silico** research has become a powerful tool in modern genetic studies, offering an efficient way to simulate complex biological systems and predict the effects of various interventions or mutations. These computer-based methods are essential for large-scale **genomic analyses** and **genetic modelling** studies, enabling researchers to rapidly explore potential outcomes that would be time-consuming or costly using traditional methods like **in vivo** or **in vitro** experiments.

In genetic modelling, **in silico** approaches can simulate gene interactions, predict the phenotypic outcomes of mutations, and even assist in the development of new therapies or drug targets based on genetic data [2].

Correct Answer: D) In silico

## References


1. Freitas AA, de Carvalho AC. A tutorial on hierarchical classification with applications in bioinformatics. Brief Bioinform. 2020;21(3):509-523.

2.  Liao B, Zhang J. In silico biology and computational modeling in bioengineering and regenerative medicine. J Biomed Res. 2019;33(4):233-242.

---

## Case 61: Calculating the Impact Factor of a Journal

### Clinical Scenario

A scientific journal received **200 citations** in the year 2023 for articles it published over the previous two years (2021 and 2022). During those two years, the journal published **50 articles** in 2021 and **25 articles** in 2022. The editor wants to calculate the **impact factor** of the journal.

### Question

What is the **impact factor** of the journal based on the provided data?

A) 1.75
B) 2.00
C) 2.66
D) 3.00
E) 4.00

### Explanation

The **impact factor** of a journal is a metric used to evaluate its influence or impact based on how often its articles are cited. The formula for calculating the impact factor is:

Impact Factor=Number of Citations in a Year/Number of Articles Published in the Previous Two Years

In this case:

- **Number of citations** in 2023 = 200

- **Number of articles** published in 2021 = 50

- **Number of articles** published in 2022 = 25

Impact Factor=200/50+25=2.66

Therefore, the impact factor of the journal is **2.66**.

### Advanced Surgical Talk

The **impact factor** is widely used as a measure of the relative importance of a scientific journal within its field. Journals with

**higher impact factors** are generally considered more influential due to their higher citation rates. However, the impact factor can sometimes be influenced by various factors, including the field of research (e.g., certain disciplines naturally receive more citations than others) and the number of articles published.

While the impact factor is useful, it is only one metric and should be interpreted alongside other measures of journal quality, such as the **h-index** or **SCImago Journal Rank (SJR)** [1][2].

Correct Answer: C) 2.66

### References

1.  Garfield E. The history and meaning of the journal impact factor. JAMA. 2006;295(1):90-93.

2.  Van Noorden R. The impact factor and other metrics: a Q&A. Nature. 2010.

---

## Case 62: Reporting Central Tendency in the Presence of Outliers

### Clinical Scenario

A hospital is reviewing the length of stay for a group of 10 postoperative patients. Most patients stayed between 2 and 5 days, but one patient had complications and stayed for **30 days**. The hospital reports the **mean** length of stay for the group, which is significantly influenced by the patient with the extended stay. The clinical team questions whether this is the best way to report the data.

### Question

Which of the following is the **most appropriate** way to report the average length of stay, considering the presence of an outlier?

A) Mean
B) Mode
C) Median
D) Range
E) Frequencies

### Explanation

The **mean** is the arithmetic average, and it is highly **susceptible to outliers**. In this case, the patient who stayed for **30 days** is an outlier that significantly **elevates the mean**, making it less representative of the typical patient's length of stay.

In situations where outliers are present, **median** (the middle value when data is ordered) or **mode** (the most frequently occurring value) are often better measures of central tendency. The **median** is particularly useful in this context because it is **not affected by outliers** and provides a more **accurate reflection of the typical length of stay**. Reporting **frequencies** (counts of how often each value occurs) is essentially the same as reporting the **mode**, which could also be appropriate.

Therefore, the **median** or **mode** is a more appropriate way to report the data than the **mean**.

### Advanced Surgical Talk

In statistical reporting, the choice of how to represent **central tendency** is crucial, especially when dealing with **outliers** that can skew the data. The **mean** is highly sensitive to outliers and may misrepresent the typical value in datasets with extreme values. The **median** is often preferred in these cases because it reflects the **middle point** of the data, giving a better sense of the central value.

For example, in a dataset where most patients stayed for **2-5 days**, but one patient stayed for **30 days**, the median would provide a **more accurate measure** of the central tendency than the mean, which would be disproportionately affected by the long stay.

Correct Answer: C) Median

### References

1. Altman DG, Bland JM. Statistics notes: The normal distribution. BMJ. 1995;310:298.

2. Wright DB. The Role of the Mean, Median, and Mode in Assessing Central Tendency in Data. Psychol Methods. 2003;8(1):87-98.

## Case 63: Choosing the Appropriate Plot for Non-Parametric Data with Outliers

### Clinical Scenario

A research team is analysing patient recovery times following surgery. The data includes several **outliers**, with most patients recovering within 5-10 days but a few requiring more than 30 days.

The distribution of the data is **non-parametric**, meaning it does not follow a normal distribution. The team needs to choose the best way to visually present the data while highlighting the outliers.

## Question

Which of the following is the most appropriate way to visually present **non-parametric data with outliers**?

A) Funnel plot
B) Forest plot
C) Scatter plot
D) Box and whisker plot
E) Bar chart

## Explanation

A **box and whisker plot** is the most suitable way to present **non-parametric data with outliers**. This type of plot displays the **median, interquartile range (IQR)**, and **outliers** in a dataset, giving a clear representation of the spread of the data, including its **skewness** and any extreme values. The box shows the middle 50% of the data (IQR), while the "whiskers" extend to the lowest and highest values within 1.5 times the IQR. Outliers are plotted as individual points beyond the whiskers, making them easy to identify.

- A **funnel plot** is used in **meta-analyses** to assess publication bias.

- A **forest plot** is used to display results of **meta-analyses** and show the effect sizes of individual studies.

- A **scatter plot** is used to display relationships between two continuous variables, but it does not specifically highlight outliers or show distribution.

- A **bar chart** is typically used to represent categorical data and is not ideal for continuous or non-parametric data with outliers.

## Advanced Surgical Talk

When analysing **non-parametric data**, especially data that contains **outliers**, it is essential to choose a visualization method that can convey the central tendency, spread, and distribution of the data clearly. The **box and whisker plot** is particularly useful for this purpose because it provides a comprehensive overview of the dataset, including:

- **Median** (the central line in the box)

- **Interquartile range (IQR)** (the box itself)

- **Outliers** (plotted as individual points beyond the whiskers)

This plot allows researchers to easily identify outliers and understand the skewness or spread of the data, making it more meaningful for **non-parametric datasets**. The **box and whisker plot** is often used in clinical research to present data that does not fit a normal distribution, especially in studies involving **continuous data** with significant variability [1][2].

**Correct Answer: D) Box and whisker plot**

**References**

1. McGill R, Tukey JW, Larsen WA. Variations of box plots. The American Statistician. 1978;32(1):12-16.

2. Bland JM, Altman DG. Statistics notes: the use of transformation when comparing two means. BMJ. 1996;312(7039):1153.

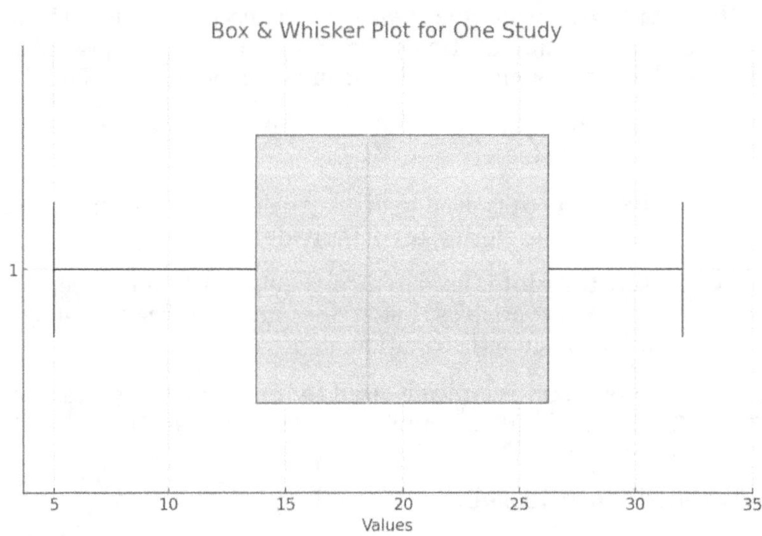


*Figure 1: Box and whisker plot*

## Clinical Scenario

A 55-year-old woman undergoes a **parathyroidectomy** for hyperparathyroidism. Postoperatively, she begins to experience **numbness and tingling** in her fingers and around her mouth, as well as muscle cramps. Blood tests reveal a significant drop in her **serum calcium levels**.

## Question

What is the most likely postoperative complication this patient is experiencing?

A) Hyperkalaemia
B) Hypocalcaemia
C) Hypercalcemia
D) Hypokalaemia
E) Hyponatremia

## Explanation

After **parathyroidectomy**, **hypocalcaemia** is a common postoperative complication, typically due to a **rebound drop in calcium levels** after the removal of hyperactive parathyroid glands. The parathyroid glands regulate calcium homeostasis by secreting **parathyroid hormone (PTH)**, which increases calcium levels in the blood. When an overactive parathyroid gland is removed, calcium levels can **drop rapidly**, leading to symptoms of **hypocalcaemia**, such as numbness, tingling, and muscle cramps.

Hypocalcaemia should be anticipated and **monitored** after parathyroidectomy, and patients may require **calcium supplementation** to manage this condition in the early postoperative period.

## Advanced Surgical Talk

**Hypocalcaemia** is one of the most common complications following **parathyroid surgery**. When the overproducing parathyroid glands are removed, the sudden decrease in **parathyroid hormone (PTH)** can lead to a rapid **decline in calcium levels**. This drop can manifest as **paraesthesia, muscle cramps, tetany**, and, in severe cases, **seizures** or **cardiac arrhythmias**.

It is important to monitor **serum calcium** levels closely after parathyroidectomy. Most cases of postoperative hypocalcaemia are

**transient**, but some patients may require **long-term calcium** and **vitamin D supplementation** to prevent prolonged symptoms. Early identification and treatment of hypocalcaemia can prevent severe complications and improve patient recovery [1][2].

**Correct Answer: B) Hypocalcaemia**

**References**

1.  Asari R, Passler C, Kaczirek K, et al. Hypoparathyroidism after total parathyroidectomy with autotransplantation in patients with renal hyperparathyroidism. Eur J Surg. 2001;167(4):296-301.

2.  Khan AA, Hanley DA, Rizzoli R, et al. Primary hyperparathyroidism: Review and recommendations on evaluation, diagnosis, and management. J Clin Endocrinol Metab. 2017;102(3):404-414.

## Case 65: Overwhelming Post-Splenectomy Infection

### Clinical Scenario

A 40-year-old man, who underwent a **splenectomy** several months ago following a traumatic injury, presents to the emergency department with high fever, confusion, and signs of sepsis. Blood tests reveal **elevated D-dimer levels**, and the patient is diagnosed with **disseminated intravascular coagulation (DIC)**.

### Question

What is the most likely diagnosis in this patient, considering his recent splenectomy and current symptoms?

A) Deep vein thrombosis
B) Pulmonary embolism
C) Overwhelming post-splenectomy infection (OPSI)
D) Sepsis from an unrelated infection
E) Haemolytic anaemia

### Explanation

The most likely diagnosis in this patient is **overwhelming post-splenectomy infection (OPSI)**, a life-threatening complication that can occur in patients who have had their spleen removed. The spleen plays a critical role in filtering bacteria and producing immune responses against encapsulated organisms (e.g., Streptococcus pneumoniae, Haemophilus influenzae, Neisseria meningitidis). Without a spleen, patients are more susceptible to overwhelming infections.

**OPSI** is characterized by rapid progression to **sepsis**, **disseminated intravascular coagulation (DIC)**, and **multi-organ failure**. The **elevated D-dimer** levels in this case are a marker of DIC, which is commonly associated with OPSI. It is critical to recognize this condition early and initiate aggressive treatment, including antibiotics and supportive care, to reduce mortality [1].

### Advanced Surgical Talk

**Overwhelming post-splenectomy infection (OPSI)** is a serious and rapid-onset infection that can occur in patients after splenectomy. It is caused by encapsulated bacteria, and patients who have had their spleen removed are at high risk due to the loss of splenic immune function. **DIC** often complicates the clinical picture, leading to widespread coagulation abnormalities and elevated **D-dimer** levels, as seen in this case.

Patients who have undergone splenectomy should be vaccinated against encapsulated organisms and educated about the risk of OPSI. They should seek immediate medical attention if they develop signs of infection. Prophylactic antibiotics are also sometimes recommended in certain high-risk patients [2].

**Correct Answer: C) Overwhelming post-splenectomy infection (OPSI)**

### References


1.  Bisharat N, Omari H, Lavi I, Raz R. Risk of infection and death among post-splenectomy patients. J Infect. 2001;43(3):182-186.

2.  Davies JM, Lewis MP, Wimperis J, et al. Review of guidelines for the prevention and treatment of infection in patients with an absent or dysfunctional spleen. Clin Med. 2011;11(5):440-443.


## Case 66: Blood Transfusion Reactions

### Clinical Scenario

A 55-year-old man receives a blood transfusion during surgery. Shortly after the transfusion, he develops shortness of breath, hypoxemia, and bilateral infiltrates on a chest X-ray. The clinical team suspects a transfusion reaction and is working to determine the underlying cause.

## Question

Which of the following is the most likely diagnosis for this patient's post-transfusion complication?

A) Transfusion-related acute lung injury (TRALI)
B) ABO incompatibility
C) Pyrexia
D) Hyperkalaemia
E) Urticaria

## Explanation

The patient's symptoms of **shortness of breath**, **hypoxemia**, and **bilateral pulmonary infiltrates** after a transfusion suggest **Transfusion-Related Acute Lung Injury (TRALI)**. **TRALI** is a rare but serious complication of blood transfusion, characterized by **acute lung injury** and non-cardiogenic pulmonary oedema within 6 hours of transfusion. It is thought to result from an immune reaction to donor antibodies targeting recipient leukocytes in the lungs, leading to capillary leakage and fluid accumulation in the alveoli.

- **ABO incompatibility** typically causes acute haemolytic reactions with fever, back pain, and haemoglobinuria.

- **Pyrexia** can occur with mild transfusion reactions but does not usually lead to severe respiratory symptoms.

- **Hyperkalaemia** is a metabolic complication of transfusion due to the breakdown of red blood cells and potassium release but presents with cardiac symptoms rather than respiratory distress.

- **Urticaria** presents as an allergic reaction with skin manifestations such as hives, but it is not associated with lung injury or hypoxemia.

## Advanced Surgical Talk

**TRALI** is one of the leading causes of transfusion-related mortality. It is characterized by the sudden onset of **hypoxemia** and **bilateral pulmonary infiltrates** within hours of a transfusion. The underlying mechanism is thought to involve donor antibodies that activate the recipient's neutrophils, leading to an inflammatory response in the lungs and causing capillary leakage and fluid buildup in the alveolar spaces.

Early recognition and supportive care, including oxygen therapy and ventilation if necessary, are essential to managing **TRALI**. Unlike other transfusion-related complications, TRALI is a non-cardiogenic cause of pulmonary oedema and should be distinguished from **transfusion-associated circulatory overload (TACO)**, which is due to fluid overload and presents with cardiac signs [1][2].

**Correct Answer: A) Transfusion-related acute lung injury (TRALI)**

### References


1.  Toy P, Popovsky MA, Abraham E, et al. Transfusion-related acute lung injury: definition and review. Crit Care Med. 2005;33(4):721-726.

2.  Rana R, Fernandez-Perez ER, Khan SA, et al. Transfusion-related acute lung injury and pulmonary edema in critically ill patients: a retrospective study. Chest. 2006;130(4):1129-113


---

## Case 67: Interpretation of Hepatitis B Serology

### Clinical Scenario

A 35-year-old woman presents for a routine health check, and her blood tests include **hepatitis B serology**. The results show the following:

- **Hepatitis B surface antigen (HBsAg)**: Negative

- **Hepatitis B surface antibody (anti-HBs)**: Positive

- **Hepatitis B core antibody (anti-HBc)**: Negative

The clinician reviews the results to determine her hepatitis B status.

### Question

What is the most likely interpretation of this patient's hepatitis B serology?

A) They are immune from hepatitis B due to vaccination
B) They are immune from hepatitis B due to previous infection
C) They are acutely infected with hepatitis B
D) They are chronically infected with hepatitis B
E) They have a resolving hepatitis B infection

## Explanation

The patient's serology shows a **positive hepatitis B surface antibody (anti-HBs)** and a **negative hepatitis B core antibody (anti-HBc)**. This pattern is consistent with **immunity due to vaccination**. After vaccination, individuals develop antibodies against the hepatitis B surface antigen (anti-HBs) without developing antibodies to the core (anti-HBc), as the core antigen is not included in the vaccine.

- **Immunity from previous infection** would show a **positive anti-HBs** and **positive anti-HBc** (due to exposure to the actual virus, which includes both surface and core antigens).

- **Acute or chronic infection** would show a **positive HBsAg**.

- A **resolving infection** would show **anti-HBs, anti-HBc**, and potentially low levels of HBsAg.

## Advanced Surgical Talk

**Hepatitis B serology** is critical in determining a patient's immune status, infection, or prior exposure to the virus. The typical interpretation of serologic markers includes:

- **HBsAg** (Hepatitis B surface antigen): Indicates active infection (acute or chronic).

- **Anti-HBs** (Hepatitis B surface antibody): Indicates immunity, either from past infection or vaccination.

- **Anti-HBc** (Hepatitis B core antibody): Indicates previous or current infection with hepatitis B.

In this case, the **positive anti-HBs** and **negative anti-HBc** suggest that the patient has been vaccinated and has developed immunity without prior infection. Hepatitis B vaccination produces immunity by generating antibodies to the surface antigen, but without exposure to the core antigen, there is no **anti-HBc** response [1][2].

**Correct Answer: A) They are immune from hepatitis B due to vaccination**

## References

1. Lok AS, McMahon BJ. **Chronic Hepatitis B: Update 2009**. Hepatology. 2009;50(3):661-662.

2.  Terrault NA, Bzowej NH, Chang KM, et al. **AASLD guidelines for treatment of chronic hepatitis B**. Hepatology. 2016;63(1):261-283.

## Case 68: Haemophilia A and Rectal Bleeding

### Clinical Scenario

A 22-year-old man with known **haemophilia A** presents to the emergency department with **rectal bleeding**. On examination, he is hemodynamically stable but has a significantly prolonged activated partial thromboplastin time (aPTT). The clinical team discusses the most appropriate treatment to manage his bleeding episode.

### Question

Which of the following is the most appropriate treatment for this patient's bleeding episode?

A) Factor VII
B) Cryoprecipitate
C) Von Willebrand factor
D) Factor V
E) Fresh frozen plasma

### Explanation

**Haemophilia A** is a genetic bleeding disorder caused by a deficiency in **Factor VIII**. Patients with haemophilia A are prone to spontaneous bleeding or bleeding following minor trauma, often in joints or soft tissues, and in this case, rectal bleeding. The treatment of choice for haemophilia A bleeding episodes is **Factor VIII replacement therapy**.

- **Factor VII**: This is used for **haemophilia B** (Factor IX deficiency) or as part of **recombinant activated Factor VII** in certain bleeding disorders, but it is not indicated for haemophilia A.

- **Cryoprecipitate**: Contains **Factor VIII, fibrinogen, von Willebrand factor**, and **Factor XIII**, but modern treatment for haemophilia A primarily involves **Factor VIII concentrates**.

- **Von Willebrand factor**: Used for **von Willebrand disease**, not haemophilia A.

- **Factor V**: Not related to haemophilia A management.

- **Fresh frozen plasma**: Contains clotting factors but is not the first-line treatment for haemophilia A due to the availability of more specific **Factor VIII concentrates**.

## Advanced Surgical Talk

**Haemophilia A** is treated by replacing the missing **Factor VIII** to control or prevent bleeding episodes. In cases of severe bleeding, like rectal bleeding in this scenario, immediate **Factor VIII replacement therapy** is crucial. If **Factor VIII concentrates** are unavailable, **cryoprecipitate**, which contains **Factor VIII**, is an alternative option. It is critical to administer the appropriate clotting factor early to prevent complications like ongoing bleeding or the development of inhibitors.

Other supportive measures, such as antifibrinolytic agents (e.g., tranexamic acid), may also be used in managing mucosal bleeding, such as rectal bleeding, in haemophilia patients [1][2].

## Correct Answer: B) Cryoprecipitate

## References


1. Srivastava A, Brewer AK, Mauser-Bunschoten EP, et al. Guidelines for the management of hemophilia. Haemophilia. 2013;19(1).

2. White GC, Rosendaal F, Aledort LM, et al. Definitions in hemophilia. Recommendation of the scientific subcommittee on factor VIII and factor IX of the ISTH. Thromb Haemost. 2001;85(3):560


---

## Case 69: Interpreting Statistical Significance

### Clinical Scenario

A clinical trial is conducted to compare the outcomes of **open Nissen fundoplication** versus **laparoscopic Nissen fundoplication** for the treatment of gastroesophageal reflux disease (GERD). The trial reports a **p-value** of **0.01**. The researchers want to interpret this result in the context of statistical significance.

# Question

What is the correct interpretation of the **p-value of 0.01** in this trial comparing open and laparoscopic Nissen fundoplication?

A) The difference is not significant
B) The threshold of significance is 90%
C) The result obtained would occur in 1% by random chance alone
D) The result shows that open Nissen fundoplication is superior to laparoscopic procedures
E) In 1% of cases, Nissen fundoplication is performed better in laparoscopic procedures compared with open

# Explanation

The **p-value** is a statistical measure that indicates the probability of observing the result, or something more extreme, if the null hypothesis is true (i.e., if there is no real difference between the groups being compared). In this case, a **p-value of 0.01** means that there is a **1% probability** that the observed difference between **open** and **laparoscopic Nissen fundoplication** outcomes occurred by **random chance alone**.

This result suggests that the difference between the two procedures is **statistically significant** at the conventional threshold of $p < 0.05$, meaning it is unlikely that the result is due to chance. However, statistical significance does not automatically imply that one procedure is **clinically superior** to the other without further analysis of effect size and clinical relevance.

- **Option C** is the correct interpretation, as a p-value of 0.01 means that there is a 1% chance that the result occurred due to random variation alone.

- **Option A** is incorrect because the result is statistically significant at $p < 0.05$.

- **Option B** is incorrect, as the conventional threshold for significance is usually 95% ($p < 0.05$), not 90%.

- **Option D** and **E** are incorrect because the p-value does not imply clinical superiority or performance—it only addresses the probability of the result occurring by chance.

# Advanced Surgical Talk

In clinical trials, the **p-value** helps determine whether the differences observed between groups are due to **random chance** or if they are likely to be **statistically significant**. In this scenario, a **p-value of 0.01** indicates that the likelihood of observing this difference by chance is 1%, which supports the conclusion that the difference is **unlikely** to be random. However, clinical interpretation requires careful consideration of **effect size**, **confidence intervals**, and **clinical outcomes**.

While the p-value can tell us if the difference is statistically significant, it does not tell us whether the difference is **clinically important**. Therefore, in addition to statistical significance, clinical significance and effect size should be evaluated when interpreting trial results [1][2].

**Correct Answer: C) The result obtained would occur in 1% by random chance alone**

### References

1.  Sterne JA, Smith GD. Sifting the evidence—what's wrong with significance tests? BMJ. 2001;322(7280):226-231.

2.  Wasserstein RL, Lazar NA. The ASA's statement on p-values: context, process, and purpose. Am Stat. 2016;70(2):129-133.

---

## Case 70: Understanding the Use of Forest Plots

### Clinical Scenario

A research team is conducting a **meta-analysis** to compare the efficacy of several treatments for a particular disease. They want to visually summarize the results from multiple studies, showing the individual effect sizes and the overall combined effect size. The figure they use shows **horizontal lines** representing the confidence intervals of the studies, with a central point estimate for each study.

### Question

Which type of plot is most appropriate for displaying the results of a **meta-analysis**?

A) ROC curve
B) Funnel plot
C) Scatter plot
D) Forest plot
E) Kaplan-Meier curve

## Explanation

A **forest plot** is the most appropriate plot for visually summarizing the results of a **meta-analysis**. It is used to display the individual study estimates of treatment effects along with their **confidence intervals**. Each study is represented by a line (indicating the confidence interval) and a central point (representing the effect estimate). The overall pooled estimate is shown at the bottom of the plot, usually as a **diamond shape** ( Figure 2).

- A **ROC curve** (Receiver Operating Characteristic) is used in **diagnostic studies** to assess the trade-off between sensitivity and specificity at various threshold levels.

- A **funnel plot** is used to assess **publication bias** in meta-analyses.

- A **scatter plot** shows the relationship between two continuous variables but is not used in meta-analysis.

- A **Kaplan-Meier curve** is used to estimate **survival probabilities** over time.

## Advanced Surgical Talk

**Forest plots** are essential in **meta-analyses** because they allow researchers to quickly assess the results of individual studies as well as the overall pooled effect. They show the degree of variation between studies (heterogeneity) and provide a clear visual representation of how different studies contribute to the overall finding. Forest plots are critical in evidence-based medicine to combine data from multiple clinical trials and assess the overall efficacy of treatments or interventions [1][2].

- **ROC curves** are often used in **diagnostic studies** to evaluate the accuracy of a diagnostic test by plotting sensitivity versus 1-specificity across different threshold values [1].

- **Funnel plots** are used to detect **publication bias** in meta-analyses by examining the distribution of study results; asymmetry in the plot may suggest bias [2].

**Correct Answer: D) Forest plot**

## References

1. Deeks JJ, Altman DG. Diagnostic tests 4: likelihood ratios. BMJ. 2004;329(7458):168-169.

2. Higgins JP, Thompson SG, Deeks JJ, Altman DG. Measuring inconsistency in meta-analyses. BMJ. 2003;327(7414):557-560.

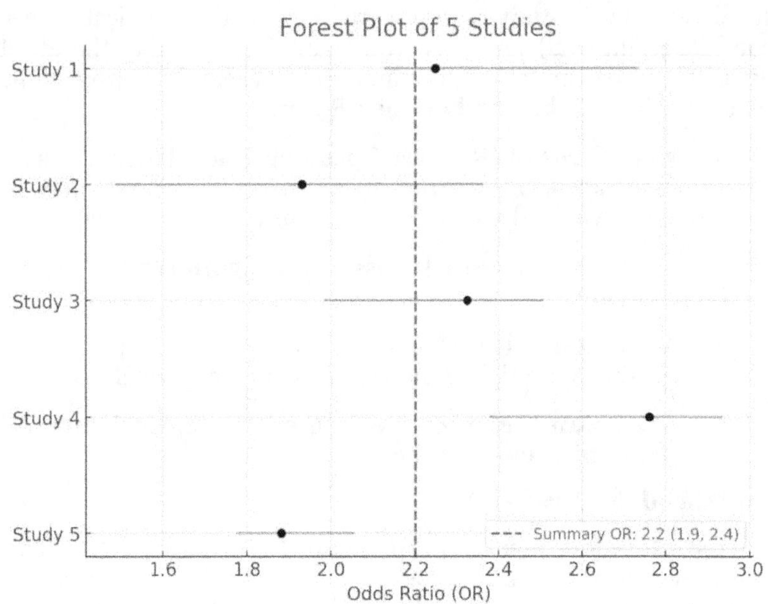


*Figure 2: Forest Plots (Blobbograms)*

## Case 71: Understanding Forest Plots (Blobbograms)

### Clinical Scenario

A group of researchers is conducting a **meta-analysis** to assess the efficacy of a new treatment compared to standard care across multiple randomized controlled trials. To visually summarize the results of these trials, they use a **forest plot**, also known as a **blobbogram**.

### Question

Which of the following statements best describes a **forest plot (blobbogram)**?

A) A plot used to assess publication bias in meta-analyses
B) A plot used to display individual study estimates and overall results in a meta-analysis

C) A plot used to compare survival rates over time
D) A plot used to display diagnostic accuracy (sensitivity and specificity)
E) A plot used to show the relationship between two continuous variables

**Explanation**

A **forest plot** (also called a **blobbogram**) is a graphical display used in **meta-analyses** to visually present the results of several studies that address the same research question. Each line in the forest plot represents an individual study's estimate of effect size, along with a **confidence interval** (usually a horizontal line). A central point or "blob" represents the **effect estimate** for each study, and the overall pooled effect estimate is typically represented as a **diamond** at the bottom of the plot.

This plot was initially developed for use in **medical research** to graphically represent the results of randomized controlled trials (RCTs). In recent years, similar **meta-analytical techniques** have been applied in **observational studies**, such as environmental epidemiology, where forest plots are also used to present results [1].

- A **funnel plot** is used to assess **publication bias** in meta-analyses.

- A **Kaplan-Meier plot** is used to compare survival rates over time.

- An **ROC curve** is used to display diagnostic accuracy by plotting sensitivity versus 1-specificity.

- A **scatter plot** shows the relationship between two continuous variables but is not used for meta-analysis.

**Advanced Surgical Talk**

The **forest plot** (blobbogram) is a powerful tool in **meta-analysis** because it visually summarizes the evidence from multiple studies, helping researchers and clinicians quickly assess the consistency and magnitude of effects across studies. Each study's result is shown as a **point estimate** (the blob) with an associated **confidence interval** (the line), while the overall pooled result is displayed as a diamond at the bottom. This visual format allows for easy comparison of individual study outcomes and the overall effect (Figure 2).

Forest plots are used not only in **randomized controlled trials** but also in **observational studies** like those in **environmental**

**epidemiology**, further broadening their utility in scientific research [2][3].

**Correct Answer: B) A plot used to display individual study estimates and overall results in a meta-analysis**

### References

1. Lewis S, Clarke M. Forest plots: trying to see the wood and the trees. BMJ. 2001;322(7300):1479-1480.

2. Higgins JP, Thompson SG, Deeks JJ, Altman DG. Measuring inconsistency in meta-analyses. BMJ. 2003;327(7414):557-560.

3. Egger M, Davey Smith G, Schneider M, Minder C. Bias in meta-analysis detected by a simple, graphical test. BMJ. 1997;315(7109):629-634.

## Case 72: Funnel Plots and Publication Bias

### Clinical Scenario

A research team is conducting a **systematic review and meta-analysis** on the effectiveness of a new medication. After compiling the results from several studies, they notice that smaller studies tend to show more positive results, while larger studies show more neutral outcomes. To investigate whether this could be due to **publication bias**, the team decides to create a **funnel plot**.

### Question

What is the purpose of a **funnel plot** in systematic reviews and meta-analyses?

A) To assess the diagnostic accuracy of a test
B) To display individual study estimates and overall results in a meta-analysis
C) To compare survival rates over time
D) To check for the existence of **publication bias**
E) To show the relationship between two continuous variables

### Explanation

A **funnel plot** is a graphical tool used to check for the presence of **publication bias** in **systematic reviews** and **meta-analyses**. In the absence of bias, the plot should resemble a **funnel shape**, with larger studies (higher precision) clustered near the average effect size and smaller studies (lower precision) spread evenly on both sides of the average. If there is a **deviation from this funnel shape**, it may indicate publication bias, where smaller studies with negative or non-significant results may be less likely to be published or included in the analysis (Figure 3).

- A **ROC curve** is used to evaluate diagnostic accuracy by plotting sensitivity and specificity.

- A **forest plot** is used to display individual study estimates and overall results in a meta-analysis.

- A **Kaplan-Meier curve** is used to compare survival rates over time.

- A **scatter plot** shows the relationship between two continuous variables but is not related to publication bias.

**Advanced Surgical Talk**

**Publication bias** is a major concern in **systematic reviews** and **meta-analyses** because studies with significant or positive findings are more likely to be published than those with negative or null results. This can skew the overall results of a meta-analysis, leading to overestimation of treatment effects.

The **funnel plot** helps detect **asymmetry** in the distribution of studies around the average effect size. If the plot is asymmetrical, with more small studies showing positive effects, it may suggest that studies with negative results have not been published or included in the analysis. This can alert researchers to potential **bias** and prompt further investigation [1][2].

Correct Answer: D) To check for the existence of publication bias

**References**


1. Sterne JA, Egger M, Davey Smith G. Systematic reviews in health care: Investigating and dealing with publication and other biases in meta-analysis. BMJ. 2001;323(7304):101-105.

2. Duval S, Tweedie R. Trim and fill: A simple funnel-plot-based method of testing and adjusting for publication bias in meta-analysis. Biometrics. 2000;56(2):455-463

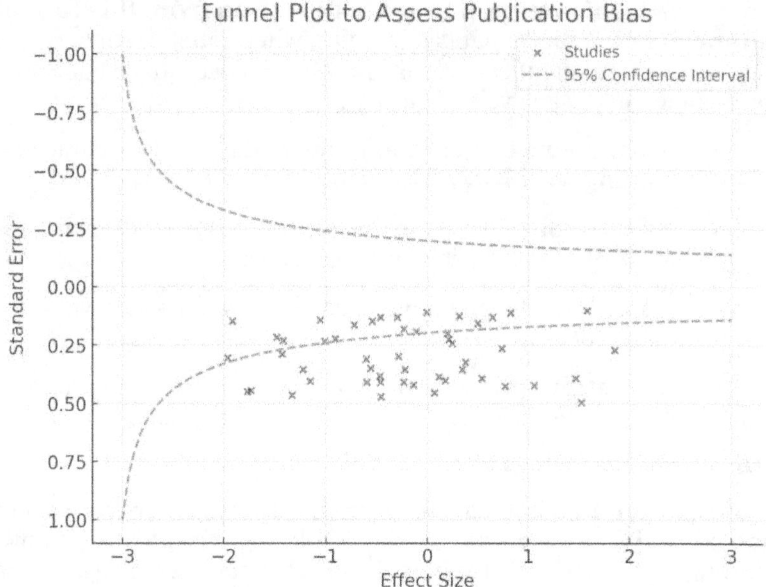


*Figure 3: Funnel Plot*

## Case 73: ROC Curves in Diagnostic Testing

### Clinical Scenario

A clinical team is evaluating a new diagnostic test for detecting early-stage cancer. They want to assess the test's ability to correctly classify patients with and without the disease by adjusting the threshold for a positive test result. To do this, they create a **Receiver Operating Characteristic (ROC) curve**.

### Question

What does the **ROC curve** illustrate in diagnostic testing?

A) The overall accuracy of the test based on the number of false positives
B) The relationship between sensitivity and specificity as the test's threshold is varied
C) The probability of a test giving a false negative result
D) The distribution of diagnostic test results for a continuous variable

E) The relationship between the number of true positives and false negatives

## Explanation

A **Receiver Operating Characteristic (ROC) curve** is a plot that illustrates the **diagnostic ability** of a binary classifier system as the **discrimination threshold** is varied. The **y-axis** represents **sensitivity** (true positive rate), while the **x-axis** represents 1 - **specificity** (false positive rate). By plotting this curve, clinicians can visualize how changes in the **threshold** for a positive test affect the balance between **sensitivity** and **specificity**.

- As the threshold for a positive test result is lowered, **sensitivity** increases (more true positives are identified), but this may come at the cost of **specificity** (more false positives).

- The **area under the ROC curve (AUC)** provides an overall measure of the test's **discriminatory power**: a perfect test has an AUC of 1.0, while a test with no discriminatory ability has an AUC of 0.5.

ROC curves are commonly used to assess the **performance** of diagnostic tests, especially when determining the optimal threshold that balances **sensitivity** and **specificity** ( Figure 4).

## Advanced Surgical Talk

The **ROC curve** is a powerful tool for evaluating the performance of **binary classification systems** like diagnostic tests. It allows clinicians and researchers to visualize how well a test can distinguish between patients with and without a condition across a range of thresholds. The **area under the curve (AUC)** is often used as a single summary statistic to compare different tests: higher AUC values indicate better diagnostic performance.

ROC curves are particularly useful when there is no clear optimal threshold, and the clinician needs to make a trade-off between **sensitivity** (catching all true cases) and **specificity** (avoiding false positives) depending on the clinical context [1][2].

Correct Answer: B) The relationship between sensitivity and specificity as the test's threshold is varied

## References

1. Fawcett T. An introduction to ROC analysis. Pattern Recognit Lett. 2006;27(8):861-874.

2.  Hanley JA, McNeil BJ. The meaning and use of the area under a receiver operating characteristic (ROC) curve. Radiology. 1982;143(1):29-36.

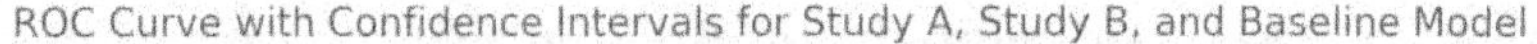

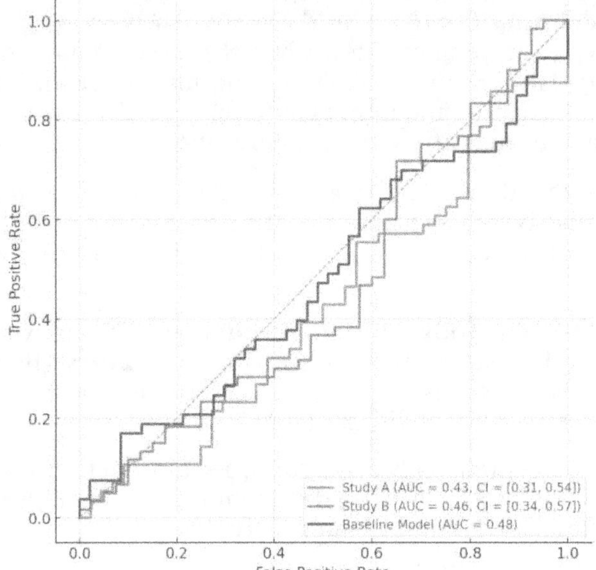



*Figure 4: Receiver Operating Characteristic (ROC) curve*

## Case 74: Funnel Plots and Publication Bias

### Clinical Scenario

A research team is conducting a **meta-analysis** on the efficacy of a new treatment. After including 7 studies, they are concerned about the possibility of **publication bias** and consider using a **funnel plot** to assess it. However, they are unsure if this method is reliable given the small number of included studies.

### Question

What is the most appropriate course of action regarding the use of a **funnel plot** to assess publication bias in this scenario?

A) A funnel plot can reliably assess publication bias with any number of studies

B) Funnel plots are best used when 5 or more studies are included
C) Funnel plots should only be used when there are 10 or more studies in the meta-analysis
D) Publication bias cannot be assessed with fewer than 10 studies, and no comment should be made
E) A reliable assessment of publication bias can be made with fewer than 10 studies

## Explanation

**Funnel plots** are traditionally used in **meta-analyses** to assess **publication bias**, which occurs when studies with negative or non-significant results are less likely to be published, leading to a skewed representation of evidence. However, when fewer than **10 studies** are included in a meta-analysis, the reliability of the funnel plot decreases.

- **Funnel plots** are most reliable when there are **10 or more studies** in the analysis. With fewer studies, the plot may not adequately reflect the true risk of publication bias. Therefore, when fewer than 10 studies are included, a simple comment noting that publication bias **cannot be reliably assessed** or that it is likely should be made, rather than relying solely on the funnel plot.

- Using a funnel plot with fewer than 10 studies does not provide sufficient reliability, and even if no bias appears in the plot, this does not necessarily mean that publication bias is absent.

## Advanced Surgical Talk

**Publication bias** can significantly affect the results of a meta-analysis by exaggerating the effectiveness of treatments. **Funnel plots** are commonly used to detect this bias by plotting the study size (precision) against the effect size. When **10 or more studies** are included, the plot takes on a **funnel shape** if publication bias is absent. However, with fewer than 10 studies, the reliability of the funnel plot diminishes, and even an apparently symmetrical plot cannot rule out bias.

In these cases, it is more appropriate to acknowledge the potential for publication bias and state that it could not be accurately assessed. **Other methods** for detecting bias, such as statistical tests, may be more reliable with fewer studies, but the funnel plot remains the most common visual tool when sufficient studies are available [1][2].

**Correct Answer: C) Funnel plots should only be used when there are 10 or more studies in the meta-analysis**

## References

1. Sterne JA, Egger M. Funnel plots for detecting bias in meta-analysis: Guidelines on choice of axis. J Clin Epidemiol. 2001;54(10):1046-1055.

2. Egger M, Davey Smith G, Schneider M, Minder C. Bias in meta-analysis detected by a simple, graphical test. BMJ. 1997;315(7109):629-634.

## Case 75: Interpreting Random Effects Model

### Clinical Scenario

A meta-analysis is conducted to assess the effect of a treatment on **pain scores** across multiple studies. The researchers choose a **random effects model** and report a pain score with an **odds ratio (OR)** of **1.4 (95% CI 1.2-2.0)**. The decision to use a random effects model was made prior to conducting the analysis.

### Question

What is the most likely reason the researchers used a **random effects model** for their meta-analysis?

A) The studies are homogeneous
B) The studies are likely to be heterogeneous
C) Random effects models are used when there is no variability between studies
D) The results are consistent across all studies
E) A fixed effects model would have been more appropriate

### Explanation

The use of a **random effects model** in a meta-analysis suggests that there is **heterogeneity** between the studies being analyzed. A random effects model assumes that the true effect size varies between studies due to differences in study populations, interventions, or methodologies. This model accounts for both **within-study** and **between-study** variability.

- In contrast, a **fixed effects model** assumes that all studies are estimating the same true effect size, which would be appropriate if the studies were **homogeneous** with minimal variability.

- The reported **OR of 1.4 (1.2-2.0)** suggests that the treatment effect is consistent across studies, but the use of the random effects model indicates that the researchers anticipated some degree of **heterogeneity** between the studies.

**Advanced Surgical Talk**

The choice between a **fixed effects** and **random effects** model is critical in meta-analysis. **Heterogeneity** refers to variations in study outcomes due to differences in study designs, populations, or interventions. When heterogeneity is present, a **random effects model** is typically chosen because it allows for variation in the true effect size across studies, accounting for both within-study and between-study differences.

In this case, the researchers used a random effects model, indicating that the studies likely had **variable methodologies or populations** that could affect the treatment's impact on pain scores. The use of the random effects model provides a **more conservative estimate** of the overall effect, as it assumes that the true effect may differ from one study to another [1][2].

**Correct Answer: B) The studies are likely to be heterogeneous**

**References**


1. Borenstein M, Hedges LV, Higgins JP, Rothstein HR. Introduction to meta-analysis. John Wiley & Sons, 2011.

2. DerSimonian R, Laird N. Meta-analysis in clinical trials. Control Clin Trials. 1986;7(3):177-188.


---

## Case 76: Interpreting Confidence Intervals

**Clinical Scenario**

A meta-analysis of **4 studies** compares the success rates of **transversus abdominis plane (TAP) blocks** versus **patient-controlled analgesia (PCA)** in emergency laparotomies. The results show a **random effects success rate of OR 1.4 (95% CI 1.2-2.0).**

**Question**

What can be deduced about the **significance** of the result?

A) The result is insignificant
B) No comment can be made
C) The p-value is <0.05
D) The p-value is >0.05
E) The success rate is equivocal

**Explanation**

The reported **odds ratio (OR) of 1.4 (1.2-2.0)** indicates that TAP blocks are associated with a **40% greater success rate** compared to PCA. The **confidence interval (CI)** does **not cross 1**, which means that the result is statistically **significant**. In odds ratio interpretation, when the **CI includes 1**, the result would be considered **not significant** as it suggests no difference between the groups.

In this case, because the **lower bound of the CI is greater than 1 (1.2)**, it can be deduced that the **p-value** is **less than 0.05**, indicating that the result is statistically significant.

- **Option C** is correct because the CI does not cross 1, meaning the result is statistically significant, and the **p-value is likely <0.05**.

- **Option A, B**, and **D** are incorrect as the result is statistically significant.

- **Option E** is incorrect as the success rate is **not equivocal**, and TAP blocks are more successful based on the OR.

**Advanced Surgical Talk**

In a meta-analysis, the **odds ratio (OR)** is a common effect size measure used to compare outcomes between two groups. When the **confidence interval (CI)** does not include **1**, the result is statistically significant, implying that there is a meaningful difference between the groups.

The **p-value** is derived from the confidence interval, and in this case, because the **CI (1.2-2.0)** does not cross **1**, it indicates that the **p-value is less than 0.05**. This means there is **less than a 5% probability** that the observed result is due to chance, confirming the significance of the findings. When interpreting results of odds ratios, a **CI excluding 1** confirms statistical significance [1][2].

Correct Answer: C) The p-value is <0.05

**References**

1. Altman DG, Bland JM. How to obtain the confidence interval from a P value. BMJ. 2011;343.

2. Higgins JP, Thompson SG, Deeks JJ, Altman DG. Measuring inconsistency in meta-analyses. BMJ. 2003;327(7414):557-560.

## Case 77: Interpreting Mean Difference

### Clinical Scenario

A meta-analysis of **4 studies** compares the effectiveness of **transversus abdominis plane (TAP) blocks** versus **patient-controlled analgesia (PCA)** for pain management in emergency laparotomies. The results show a **mean difference in pain scores of -1.4 (95% CI -1.8 to 2.0)**.

### Question

What can be deduced about the **significance** of the result?

A) The result is insignificant
B) No comment can be made
C) The p-value is <0.05
D) The p-value is significant
E) The success rate is equivocal

### Explanation

The mean difference reported is **-1.4**, with a **95% confidence interval (CI) of -1.8 to 2.0**. In this case, the **confidence interval crosses zero** (it ranges from a negative value to a positive value). When the confidence interval includes **zero** in a meta-analysis, it means that there is no statistically significant difference between the two groups being compared, as the true effect could be **zero**.

- The fact that the confidence interval includes zero means that the result is **not statistically significant**.

- Therefore, **Option A** ("The result is insignificant") is correct.

- **Option C** and **D** are incorrect because the p-value would be **>0.05**, indicating that the result is **not significant**.

- • **Option E** is incorrect because the success rate is not the focus in this scenario, and the pain mean difference does not indicate a statistically significant result.

**Advanced Surgical Talk**

In a meta-analysis, when the **mean difference** between two interventions (TAP blocks vs PCA, in this case) is being analyzed, the **confidence interval (CI)** is key to determining the statistical significance of the result. If the CI **crosses zero**, it implies that the true difference between the interventions might be **zero**, indicating that there is no significant difference between the two treatments.

In this case, the **CI of -1.8 to 2.0** crosses zero, so the result is not statistically significant. It suggests that the TAP block may not provide significantly better or worse pain relief compared to PCA in this scenario, as the true effect might be zero [1][2].

**Correct Answer: A) The result is insignificant**

**References**

1. Altman DG, Bland JM. How to obtain the confidence interval from a P value. BMJ. 2011;343.

2. Higgins JP, Thompson SG, Deeks JJ, Altman DG. Measuring inconsistency in meta-analyses. BMJ. 2003;327(7414):557-560.

---

## Case 78: Calculating Number Needed to Treat

**Clinical Scenario**

A clinical trial is conducted to assess the effectiveness of a new drug for preventing post-operative infections. The results show that **20 out of 200 patients** in the treatment group developed an infection, while **5 out of 100 patients** in the control group developed an infection. The clinician is asked to calculate the **number needed to treat (NNT)** to prevent one additional infection.

**Question**

How is the **number needed to treat (NNT)** calculated, and what is the NNT based on the given data?

A) 5
B) 10
C) 20

D) 25
E) 50

## Explanation

The **number needed to treat (NNT)** is a measure used to indicate how many patients need to be treated with a particular intervention to prevent one additional adverse event, in this case, infection. It is calculated using the **absolute risk reduction (ARR)**, which is the difference in event rates between the control and treatment groups.

Step-by-step calculation:

1. **Event rate in the treatment group**: 20/200 = **0.10** (10%)

2. **Event rate in the control group**: 5/100 = **0.05** (5%)

Absolute Risk Reduction (ARR)=0.10−0.05=0.05 (5%)

**Number needed to treat (NNT)** is the inverse of ARR:

NNT=1/ARR=1/0.05=20

Thus, the NNT is **20**, meaning that **20 patients** need to be treated to prevent one additional infection.

## Advanced Surgical Talk

The **number needed to treat (NNT)** is a valuable metric in clinical practice because it provides a clear and practical understanding of how effective a treatment is. A lower NNT is generally preferable, as it indicates that fewer patients need to be treated to prevent one adverse event.

In this example, an NNT of **20** means that for every **20 patients treated** with the new drug, **one infection** will be prevented. NNT should always be interpreted alongside other clinical factors, such as side effects and costs, when making treatment decisions [1][2].

Correct Answer: C) 20

## References

1. McQuay HJ, Moore RA. Using numerical results from systematic reviews in clinical practice. Ann Intern Med. 1997;126(9):712-720.

2.  Laupacis A, Sackett DL, Roberts RS. An assessment of clinically useful measures of the consequences of treatment. N Engl J Med. 1988;318(26):1728-1733.

## Case 79: Synthesis Phase of the Cell Cycle

### Clinical Scenario

A medical student is learning about the **cell cycle** and its phases to better understand how cancer drugs target different stages of cell division. The student is particularly interested in the phase where **DNA replication** occurs, which is critical for understanding the action of certain **chemotherapeutic agents**.

### Question

Which phase of the cell cycle is characterized by **DNA synthesis**?

A) G0 phase
B) G1 phase
C) S phase
D) G2 phase
E) M phase

### Explanation

The **S phase** (Synthesis phase) of the cell cycle is the phase during which **DNA replication** occurs. This is a critical step in the cell cycle because the cell must duplicate its genetic material before dividing. Cancer drugs that target the **S phase** often work by interfering with **DNA synthesis**, thus preventing the cancer cells from proliferating.

- The **G0 phase** is a resting state where the cell is not actively dividing.

- The **G1 phase** is the first growth phase where the cell prepares for DNA synthesis.

- The **G2 phase** is the second growth phase where the cell prepares for mitosis.

- The **M phase** (Mitosis) is where the cell divides into two daughter cells.

Understanding the **S phase** is critical for comprehending the mechanism of action of several **chemotherapeutic agents**, such as **antimetabolites** (e.g., methotrexate and 5-fluorouracil), which specifically target this phase to prevent DNA replication in rapidly dividing cancer cells.

## Advanced Surgical Talk

The **cell cycle** is a tightly regulated process that is crucial for normal cell division and growth. **Chemotherapeutic agents** often target different phases of the cell cycle, depending on their mechanism of action. Drugs that target the **S phase** inhibit **DNA replication**, which is a key point of vulnerability for rapidly dividing cancer cells.

Understanding the role of each phase in the cell cycle helps clinicians select **targeted therapies** that disrupt cancer cell proliferation while minimizing damage to normal cells. For example, **antimetabolites** like methotrexate disrupt nucleotide synthesis, preventing cancer cells from successfully replicating their DNA during the S phase [1][2].

**Correct Answer: C) S phase**

## References

1. Vermeulen K, Van Bockstaele DR, Berneman ZN. The cell cycle: a review of regulation, deregulation and therapeutic targets in cancer. Cell Prolif. 2003;36(3):131-149.

2. Murray AW. Cell cycle checkpoints. Curr Opin Cell Biol. 1995;7(6):872-876.

---

## Case 80: Mechanism of Action of Vincristine

### Clinical Scenario

A 45-year-old woman is being treated with **vincristine** as part of her chemotherapy regimen for lymphoma. The medical team explains that vincristine works by interfering with the cancer cells' ability to divide, particularly targeting the phase of the cell cycle where **microtubules** play a critical role.

### Question

How does **vincristine** work in the treatment of cancer?

A) Prevents the breakdown of microtubules in the M phase
B) Prevents the formation of microtubules in the M phase
C) Prevents the formation of microtubules in the G2 phase
D) Impairs microtubule function in the S phase
E) Impairs microtubule function in the M phase

## Explanation

**Vincristine** is a chemotherapeutic agent that works by **preventing the formation of microtubules** during the **M phase** of the cell cycle. Microtubules are essential for the proper segregation of chromosomes during **mitosis** (M phase). By inhibiting their formation, vincristine causes cells to arrest in mitosis, leading to cell death, particularly in rapidly dividing cancer cells.

- **Option B** is correct: Vincristine acts specifically during the **M phase** to prevent the **formation of microtubules**.

- **Option A** is incorrect: Drugs like **taxanes** prevent the **breakdown** of microtubules, but vincristine inhibits their formation.

- **Option C** is incorrect: Microtubule formation is a key event in the M phase, not the G2 phase.

- **Option D** and **E** are incorrect because vincristine acts in the M phase, not the S phase.

## Advanced Surgical Talk

**Vincristine** is part of the **vinca alkaloid** class of chemotherapy agents, which exert their effects by binding to **tubulin** and inhibiting the assembly of microtubules. Microtubules are crucial for the formation of the **mitotic spindle**, which is responsible for separating chromosomes during cell division. By inhibiting microtubule formation, vincristine causes **mitotic arrest**, leading to apoptosis in rapidly dividing cells, such as cancer cells.

Vincristine is commonly used to treat various malignancies, including **leukaemias**, **lymphomas**, and **solid tumours**. Understanding its mechanism helps in anticipating side effects, such as **neurotoxicity**, which is related to its action on microtubules in nerve cells [1][2].

Correct Answer: B) Prevents the formation of microtubules in the M phase

## References


1. Jordan MA, Wilson L. Microtubules as a target for anticancer drugs. Nat Rev Cancer. 2004;4(4):253-265.

2. Dumontet C, Jordan MA. Microtubule-binding agents: A dynamic field of cancer therapeutics. Nat Rev Drug Discov. 2010;9(10):790-803.

# Case 81: Side Effects of Vincristine

## Clinical Scenario

A 60-year-old man is receiving **vincristine** as part of his chemotherapy regimen for lymphoma. During a follow-up visit, the patient reports numbness and tingling in his fingers and toes. The medical team is concerned about potential side effects from the vincristine treatment.

## Question

What is the **main concern** regarding the side effects of vincristine?

A) The main concern is neurotoxicity
B) The main concern is a dry mouth
C) The main concern is arthralgia
D) There are no major side effects
E) None of the above

## Explanation

The **main concern** with **vincristine** is **neurotoxicity**, which is its most common and significant **dose-limiting side effect**. **Neurotoxicity** can manifest as **peripheral neuropathy**, with symptoms such as numbness, tingling, weakness, and sometimes **gastrointestinal** side effects like **constipation** or **ileus**. This toxicity occurs because vincristine disrupts microtubule function, which is essential for normal nerve cell operations.

- **Option A** is correct: The most common and concerning side effect of vincristine is **neurotoxicity**.

- **Option B** (dry mouth) and **Option C** (arthralgia) are less relevant as side effects of vincristine.

- **Option D** is incorrect because vincristine has significant side effects, particularly neurotoxicity.

- **Option E** is incorrect because neurotoxicity is a major side effect.

## Advanced Surgical Talk

**Vincristine** is a potent chemotherapy drug, but its use is limited by its **neurotoxic side effects**, which can manifest as **peripheral neuropathy**. Patients may experience numbness, tingling, muscle weakness, and sometimes gastrointestinal complications like **paralytic ileus**. This occurs because vincristine interferes with

**microtubules** in nerve cells, disrupting axonal transport, which is essential for nerve function.

Neurotoxicity is a **dose-limiting** side effect, meaning that treatment doses must often be reduced to prevent further nerve damage. Monitoring patients for early signs of neurotoxicity is crucial to avoid long-term nerve damage. Other side effects like **gastrointestinal toxicity** (e.g., constipation) can also occur but are less limiting compared to neurotoxicity [1][2].

**Correct Answer: A) The main concern is neurotoxicity**

### References


1. Argyriou AA, Koltzenburg M, Polychronopoulos P, et al. Vincristine-induced peripheral neuropathy. Crit Rev Oncol Hematol. 2008;62(3):229-239.

2. Verstappen CC, Heimans JJ, Hoekman K, Postma TJ. Neurotoxic complications of chemotherapy in patients with cancer: clinical signs and optimal management. Drugs. 2003;63(15):1549-1563.


## Case 82: Mechanism of Action of Paclitaxel

### Clinical Scenario

A 48-year-old woman is receiving **paclitaxel** as part of her chemotherapy regimen for breast cancer. The oncologist explains that paclitaxel targets **microtubules**, which are crucial for cell division, particularly during the **M phase** of the cell cycle.

### Question

How does **paclitaxel** work in the treatment of cancer?

A) Prevents the breakdown of microtubules in the M phase
B) Prevents the formation of microtubules in the M phase
C) Prevents the formation of microtubules in the G2 phase
D) Prevents microtubule breakdown in the S phase
E) Impairs microtubule function in the M phase

### Explanation

**Paclitaxel** is a chemotherapeutic agent that works by **preventing the breakdown of microtubules** during the **M phase** of the cell cycle. Microtubules are essential for separating chromosomes during **mitosis**. Normally, microtubules form and disassemble to allow cell division, but paclitaxel stabilizes them, preventing their disassembly and thus **blocking cell division**.

- **Option A** is correct: Paclitaxel **prevents the breakdown of microtubules** in the **M phase**, leading to cell cycle arrest and eventual apoptosis in rapidly dividing cells.

- **Option B** is incorrect: Drugs like **vincristine** prevent the **formation** of microtubules, but paclitaxel prevents their breakdown.

- **Option C** and **Option D** are incorrect because paclitaxel acts during the M phase, not the G2 or S phase.

- **Option E** is incorrect because it does not simply impair microtubule function but specifically prevents their disassembly in the M phase.

**Advanced Surgical Talk**

**Paclitaxel** is a member of the **taxane** family of chemotherapy drugs. By preventing the disassembly of **microtubules**, paclitaxel disrupts the normal process of mitosis, leading to **mitotic arrest** and cell death, particularly in rapidly dividing cancer cells. This makes paclitaxel highly effective in treating cancers like **breast cancer** and **ovarian cancer**.

Unlike drugs like **vincristine**, which inhibit microtubule assembly, paclitaxel works by stabilizing microtubules, preventing their normal depolymerization during mitosis. This interference with the dynamic structure of microtubules is what causes the cell to arrest in the **M phase** and eventually die [1][2].

Correct Answer: A) Prevents the breakdown of microtubules in the M phase

**References**

1. Jordan MA, Wilson L. Microtubules as a target for anticancer drugs. Nat Rev Cancer. 2004;4(4):253-265.

2. Weaver BA. How Taxol/paclitaxel kills cancer cells. Mol Biol Cell. 2014;25(18):2677-2681.

## Clinical Scenario

A 55-year-old woman is receiving **paclitaxel** as part of her chemotherapy regimen for ovarian cancer. After a few treatment cycles, she reports numbness and tingling in her hands and feet, raising concerns about possible side effects of the drug.

## Question

What is the **main concern** regarding the side effects of paclitaxel?

A) The main concern is neurotoxicity
B) The main concern is neuropathy
C) The main concern is arthralgia
D) There are no major side effects
E) None of the above

## Explanation

The **main concern** with **paclitaxel** is **neuropathy**, which is a common and dose-limiting side effect. Paclitaxel can cause **peripheral neuropathy**, leading to symptoms such as numbness, tingling, and weakness, primarily in the hands and feet. This neuropathy results from damage to peripheral nerves, often manifesting after several cycles of treatment.

- **Option B** is correct: The most significant side effect of paclitaxel is **neuropathy**, which affects the patient's peripheral nerves.

- **Option A** (neurotoxicity) is a broader term, and while neuropathy is a form of neurotoxicity, the more specific concern with paclitaxel is **neuropathy**.

- **Option C** (arthralgia) is less common compared to neuropathy but can occur as a secondary side effect.

- **Option D** and **E** are incorrect because paclitaxel has significant side effects, particularly **neuropathy**.

## Advanced Surgical Talk

**Paclitaxel** is a highly effective chemotherapeutic agent, but it is associated with significant side effects, the most concerning of which is **peripheral neuropathy**. This side effect occurs due to the drug's impact on **microtubules** in nerve cells, disrupting axonal transport and causing nerve damage. The neuropathy is usually **dose-dependent** and can worsen with cumulative doses, sometimes leading to long-term nerve damage if not managed appropriately.

In addition to neuropathy, paclitaxel can cause other side effects, such as **myelosuppression, arthralgia**, and **gastrointestinal disturbances**, but neuropathy remains the most common **dose-limiting toxicity**. Early recognition and dose adjustments are crucial to prevent severe or irreversible neuropathy [1][2].

**Correct Answer: B) The main concern is neuropathy**

### References


1. Verstappen CC, Heimans JJ, Hoekman K, Postma TJ. Neurotoxic complications of chemotherapy in patients with cancer: clinical signs and optimal management. Drugs. 2003;63(15):1549-1563.

2. Scripture CD, Figg WD, Sparreboom A. Peripheral neuropathy induced by paclitaxel: recent insights and future perspectives. Curr Neuropharmacol. 2006;4(2):165-172.


## Case 84: Mechanism of Action of Eribulin

### Clinical Scenario

A 50-year-old woman is receiving **eribulin** as part of her chemotherapy regimen for metastatic breast cancer. The oncologist explains that eribulin targets **microtubules**, which are essential for cell division, particularly during the **M phase** of the cell cycle.

### Question

How does **eribulin** work in the treatment of cancer?

A) Prevents the breakdown of microtubules in the M phase
B) Prevents the formation of microtubules in the M phase
C) Prevents the formation of microtubules in the G2 phase
D) Prevents microtubule breakdown in the S phase
E) Impairs microtubule function in the M phase

### Explanation

**Eribulin** works by **binding to high-affinity ends of microtubules** and preventing their proper function, leading to disruption of the **M phase** of the cell cycle. This inhibition leads to **mitotic arrest**, which prevents cancer cells from completing cell division and leads to cell death.

- **Option B** is correct: Eribulin **prevents the formation of microtubules** in the **M phase** by binding to the ends of microtubules, thereby impairing their ability to polymerize and function properly.

- **Option A** (prevents breakdown) is incorrect because eribulin works by **inhibiting microtubule formation** rather than preventing their breakdown.

- **Option C** (G2 phase) is incorrect because eribulin targets the **M phase** of the cell cycle, not the G2 phase.

- **Option D** (S phase) is incorrect because microtubules are important in the **M phase**, not the S phase.

- **Option E** (impairs microtubule function in the M phase) is partially correct, but the most accurate description is that it **prevents the formation of microtubules**.

**Advanced Surgical Talk**

**Eribulin** is a **microtubule dynamics inhibitor** that binds to the **plus ends of microtubules**, which are critical for microtubule growth. By preventing the proper elongation of microtubules during mitosis, eribulin causes **mitotic arrest** and eventually induces apoptosis in cancer cells. Eribulin is used in the treatment of **metastatic breast cancer** and has shown efficacy in cases resistant to other microtubule-targeting agents like **taxanes**.

Eribulin's unique binding mechanism at the ends of microtubules distinguishes it from other microtubule inhibitors, which may either prevent assembly (like **vincristine**) or prevent disassembly (like **paclitaxel**). This action makes eribulin particularly effective in disrupting cancer cell division [1][2].

**Correct Answer: B) Prevents the formation of microtubules in the M phase**

**References**

1. Jordan MA, Wilson L. Microtubules as a target for anticancer drugs. Nat Rev Cancer. 2004;4(4):253-265.

2. Smith JA, Wilson L, Azarenko O, et al. Eribulin binds at microtubule ends to suppress dynamic instability and inhibit the growth of taxane-resistant cancer cells. Cancer Res. 2010;70(3):970-979.

## Clinical Scenario

A 52-year-old woman is being treated with **eribulin** for metastatic breast cancer. During follow-up visits, she complains of **joint pain** and discomfort. The medical team is monitoring for potential side effects associated with the chemotherapy.

## Question

What is the **main concern** regarding the side effects of eribulin?

A) The main concern is neurotoxicity
B) The main concern is neuropathy
C) The main concern is arthralgia
D) There are no major side effects
E) None of the above

## Explanation

The **main concern** with **eribulin** is **arthralgia**, which refers to **joint pain** and discomfort. **Arthralgia** is a common side effect of eribulin and can significantly impact a patient's quality of life during chemotherapy. Patients may report pain in various joints, which can limit mobility and daily activities.

- **Option C** is correct: **Arthralgia** is a key side effect of eribulin.

- **Option A** (neurotoxicity) and **Option B** (neuropathy) are common concerns with other microtubule inhibitors like vincristine and paclitaxel, but **arthralgia** is more commonly associated with eribulin.

- **Option D** is incorrect because eribulin does have significant side effects, especially **arthralgia**.

- **Option E** is incorrect because arthralgia is the correct concern.

## Advanced Surgical Talk

**Eribulin** is a chemotherapy agent used in treating **metastatic breast cancer**. One of its more common side effects is **arthralgia** or joint pain, which can be distressing for patients. While eribulin can also cause **neutropenia, fatigue**, and **alopecia**, joint pain is often a significant limiting factor in its use.

Managing the side effects of eribulin involves pain control strategies, including the use of **nonsteroidal anti-inflammatory drugs (NSAIDs)** or other analgesics, depending on the severity of the symptoms. **Neuropathy** and **neurotoxicity**, while important concerns with other microtubule-targeting agents like paclitaxel, are less of a concern with eribulin [1][2].

**Correct Answer: C) The main concern is arthralgia**

### References


1. Cortes J, O'Shaughnessy J, Loesch D, et al. Eribulin monotherapy versus treatment of physician's choice in patients with metastatic breast cancer (EMBRACE): a phase 3 open-label randomised study. Lancet. 2011;377(9769):914-923.

2. Twelves C, Cortes J, Vahdat L, et al. Eribulin monotherapy in patients with metastatic breast cancer: a pooled analysis of two phase 3 studies. Breast Cancer Res Treat. 2014;148(3):553-561.


## Case 86: Mechanism of Action of Cisplatin

### Clinical Scenario

A 58-year-old man with lung cancer is receiving **cisplatin** as part of his chemotherapy regimen. The oncologist explains that cisplatin works by **cross-linking DNA**, interfering with the cancer cell's ability to replicate.

### Question

How does **cisplatin** work in the treatment of cancer?

A) Works in the G2 phase and cross-links DNA
B) Cross-links DNA at Guanine in the S phase
C) Cross-links DNA in the M phase
D) Cross-links DNA in the G1 phase
E) Crosses the blood-brain barrier

### Explanation

**Cisplatin** is a chemotherapy drug that works by **cross-linking DNA**, specifically targeting **guanine** residues, which leads to the inhibition of DNA replication and transcription. Cisplatin is most effective in the **G1 phase**, where it prevents cancer cells from progressing through the cell cycle. By forming **DNA adducts**, cisplatin causes DNA damage that the cell cannot repair, ultimately leading to apoptosis (programmed cell death).

- **Option D** is correct: Cisplatin **cross-links DNA** in the **G1 phase**, preventing the cell from progressing to the next stage of the cell cycle.

- **Option A** (G2 phase) and **Option B** (S phase) are incorrect because cisplatin's primary action is in the **G1 phase**.

- **Option C** is incorrect because the M phase (mitosis) is not the primary target of cisplatin.

- **Option E** is incorrect because cisplatin does not effectively **cross the blood-brain barrier**.

**Advanced Surgical Talk**

**Cisplatin** is a platinum-based chemotherapy agent used to treat various cancers, including **lung, testicular**, and **ovarian cancers**. By **cross-linking DNA** at **guanine residues**, it forms **intrastrand and interstrand cross-links**, which inhibit DNA replication and transcription. This leads to **DNA damage** that cannot be easily repaired, pushing the cell toward apoptosis.

Cisplatin primarily acts during the **G1 phase** of the cell cycle, where it prevents the cancer cell from progressing to DNA synthesis (S phase). Its broad-spectrum efficacy makes it a cornerstone of chemotherapy, but its use is often limited by side effects, including **nephrotoxicity, ototoxicity**, and **neurotoxicity** [1][2].

Correct Answer: D) Cross-links DNA in the G1 phase

**References**

1.  Wang D, Lippard SJ. Cellular processing of platinum anticancer drugs. Nat Rev Drug Discov. 2005;4(4):307-320.

2.  Florea AM, Büsselberg D. Cisplatin as an anti-tumor drug: cellular mechanisms of activity, drug resistance and induced side effects. Cancers (Basel). 2011;3(1):1351-1371.

---

## Case 87: Side Effects of Cisplatin

### Clinical Scenario

A 60-year-old man receiving **cisplatin** as part of his chemotherapy regimen for testicular cancer develops symptoms of **hearing loss** and **nausea**. The oncologist explains that these are potential side effects of the treatment, and that kidney function also needs to be monitored closely.

## Question

What is the **main concern** regarding the side effects of cisplatin?

A) The main concern is neurotoxicity
B) The main concern is neuropathy
C) The main concern is arthralgia
D) There are no major side effects
E) The main concern is ototoxicity

## Explanation

The **main concern** with **cisplatin** is **ototoxicity**, which refers to damage to the **inner ear**, resulting in **hearing loss** or **tinnitus**. Cisplatin can also cause **nephrotoxicity**, where the kidneys are affected, leading to impaired renal function. Monitoring both kidney function and hearing is critical during cisplatin treatment.

- **Option E** is correct: **Ototoxicity** is a significant concern with cisplatin, especially in younger patients and those receiving higher doses.

- **Option A** and **B** (neurotoxicity and neuropathy) are side effects, but **nephrotoxicity** and **ototoxicity** are more commonly dose-limiting side effects.

- **Option C** (arthralgia) is not a common side effect of cisplatin.

- **Option D** is incorrect because cisplatin has several significant side effects.

## Advanced Surgical Talk

**Cisplatin** is widely used in the treatment of cancers like **testicular**, **ovarian**, and **lung cancer**, but its use is limited by several significant side effects:

- **Ototoxicity**: Cisplatin can damage the inner ear, leading to **permanent hearing loss**, which may be dose-dependent.

- **Nephrotoxicity**: Cisplatin can cause **kidney damage**, leading to acute kidney injury and electrolyte disturbances.

- **Neurotoxicity**: While **peripheral neuropathy** may occur, it is less common than the other toxicities.

- **Gastrointestinal toxicity**: Cisplatin is also associated with **nausea and vomiting**.

Regular monitoring of **renal function** and **hearing** is crucial for patients undergoing cisplatin therapy. Dose adjustments or alternative chemotherapy regimens may be considered in patients at higher risk for these side effects [1][2].

**Correct Answer: E) The main concern is ototoxicity**

**References**

1. Ruggiero A, Rizzo D, Trombatore G, et al. Evaluation of cisplatin-induced nephrotoxicity in pediatric patients treated for solid tumors. Front Pharmacol. 2017;8:503.

2. Tange RA. Ototoxicity: mechanisms and protective strategies. Clin Otolaryngol Allied Sci. 1998;23(5):370-376.

## Case 88: Cisplatin-Induced Nephrotoxicity

### Clinical Scenario

A 55-year-old man undergoing chemotherapy with **cisplatin** for lung cancer develops **acute kidney injury** with elevated creatinine levels, consistent with **cisplatin-induced nephrotoxicity**. The oncologist considers administering **amifostine** to help prevent further kidney damage.

### Question

What is the role of **amifostine** in the context of cisplatin treatment?

A) Amifostine increases the efficacy of cisplatin
B) Amifostine reverses ototoxicity caused by cisplatin
C) Amifostine is used to prevent nephrotoxicity caused by cisplatin
D) Amifostine is used to prevent neuropathy caused by cisplatin
E) Amifostine decreases cisplatin's anticancer activity

### Explanation

**Amifostine** is a cytoprotective agent used to **reduce the nephrotoxicity** associated with **cisplatin** treatment. It works by scavenging free radicals and protecting normal tissues from the toxic effects of chemotherapy, particularly in the kidneys. **Nephrotoxicity** is a significant dose-limiting side effect of cisplatin, and using amifostine can help **prevent** or **mitigate** kidney damage, while still allowing the patient to receive effective cancer treatment.

- **Option C** is correct: Amifostine is specifically used to **prevent nephrotoxicity** associated with cisplatin.

- **Option A** is incorrect: While amifostine does not increase cisplatin's efficacy, it protects normal tissues.

- **Option B** is incorrect: Amifostine does not reverse or prevent **ototoxicity** caused by cisplatin.

- **Option D** is incorrect: While **neuropathy** is a concern with cisplatin, amifostine is mainly used to protect the kidneys, not nerves.

- **Option E** is incorrect: Amifostine does not reduce the **anticancer activity** of cisplatin.

## Advanced Surgical Talk

**Cisplatin-induced nephrotoxicity** is a major concern in the treatment of cancer patients. Cisplatin can cause **acute kidney injury**, **electrolyte imbalances**, and long-term renal damage due to its toxic effects on the renal tubular cells. **Amifostine** is an FDA-approved agent that helps protect the kidneys from these effects by **neutralizing free radicals** and providing cellular protection to normal tissues.

While amifostine is effective at reducing **nephrotoxicity**, it does not prevent other side effects of cisplatin, such as **ototoxicity** or **neuropathy**. The use of amifostine allows patients to continue cisplatin therapy without compromising renal function, which is especially important in patients receiving high doses or those with pre-existing renal impairment [1][2].

**Correct Answer: C) Amifostine is used to prevent nephrotoxicity caused by cisplatin**

## References


1. Santoso JT, Lucci JA 3rd, Coleman RL, Schafer I, Hannigan EV. Amifostine: the clinical applications of a cytoprotective agent. Expert Opin Pharmacother. 2003;4(8):1349-1361.

2. Launay-Vacher V, Rey JB, Isnard-Bagnis C, et al. Prevention of cisplatin nephrotoxicity: state of the art and recommendations from the Cancer and the Kidney International Network. Kidney Int. 2008;73(7):1007-1018.

## Clinical Scenario

A 45-year-old man is receiving **cyclophosphamide** as part of his chemotherapy regimen for lymphoma. He presents with **blood in his urine**, dysuria, and abdominal pain. The oncologist suspects **haemorrhagic cystitis**, a known side effect of cyclophosphamide.

## Question

What is the recommended treatment to **prevent** or **manage** haemorrhagic cystitis caused by cyclophosphamide?

A) Amifostine
B) MESNA
C) Allopurinol
D) Furosemide
E) Dexamethasone

## Explanation

**Haemorrhagic cystitis** is a common side effect of **cyclophosphamide** due to the production of a toxic metabolite called **acrolein**, which irritates the bladder lining and causes bleeding. **MESNA** (mercaptoethane sulfonate sodium) is used to prevent this complication by binding to acrolein in the urine and neutralizing its toxic effects, thereby protecting the bladder.

- **Option B** is correct: **MESNA** is the drug used to prevent or treat **haemorrhagic cystitis** associated with cyclophosphamide use.

- **Option A** (Amifostine) is incorrect: While amifostine is used to prevent **nephrotoxicity** with cisplatin, it is not effective against haemorrhagic cystitis.

- **Option C** (Allopurinol) is used to prevent **tumour lysis syndrome**, not haemorrhagic cystitis.

- **Option D** (Furosemide) is a diuretic that helps increase urine output but does not prevent bladder toxicity.

- **Option E** (Dexamethasone) is a corticosteroid, not relevant for managing haemorrhagic cystitis.

**Advanced Surgical Talk**

**Cyclophosphamide** and other alkylating agents can cause **haemorrhagic cystitis**, which may range from mild irritation to severe bleeding. This complication arises due to the accumulation of the toxic byproduct **acrolein** in the bladder. **MESNA** is co-administered with cyclophosphamide to bind acrolein in the urine and protect the bladder lining from its harmful effects.

Cyclophosphamide treatment protocols typically include **hydration** and the use of MESNA to prevent haemorrhagic cystitis. If haemorrhagic cystitis develops, supportive treatments such as increased fluid intake and MESNA doses are often intensified [1][2].

**Correct Answer: B) MESNA**

**References**


1. Korkmaz A, Oter S, Deveci S, et al. Prevention of cyclophosphamide-induced hemorrhagic cystitis by MESNA: a review. Curr Pharm Des. 2008;14(13):1201-1206.

2. Emadi A, Jones RJ, Brodsky RA. Cyclophosphamide and cancer: golden anniversary. Nat Rev Clin Oncol. 2009;6(11):638-647.


---

## Case 90: Mechanism of Action of Capecitabine

### Clinical Scenario

A 62-year-old woman with metastatic colorectal cancer is prescribed **capecitabine** as part of her chemotherapy regimen. The oncologist explains that capecitabine is a **prodrug** that is converted into its active form in the body, targeting cancer cells by inhibiting DNA synthesis.

### Question

How does **capecitabine** work in the treatment of cancer?

A) Inhibits thymidylate synthase resulting in impaired DNA synthesis
B) Works in the G1 phase by enhancing thymidylate synthase
C) Works in the G2 phase resulting in enhanced normal DNA synthesis
D) Works in the M phase by ensuring DNA crosslinking
E) None of the above

## Explanation

**Capecitabine** is a prodrug that is converted to **5-fluorouracil (5-FU)** in the body. Its active form, 5-FU, works by **inhibiting thymidylate synthase**, an enzyme that is essential for the synthesis of **thymidine**, a building block of DNA. By inhibiting this enzyme, capecitabine causes a **block in DNA synthesis**, leading to impaired cell replication and eventual cell death. This makes capecitabine particularly effective against rapidly dividing cancer cells ( Table 6).

- **Option A** is correct: Capecitabine inhibits **thymidylate synthase**, which leads to **impaired DNA synthesis**.

- **Option B** is incorrect: Capecitabine does not enhance thymidylate synthase but inhibits it.

- **Option C** is incorrect: Capecitabine does not work in the **G2 phase**.

- **Option D** is incorrect: Capecitabine does not work by crosslinking DNA in the M phase.

## Advanced Surgical Talk

**Capecitabine** is a widely used oral chemotherapeutic agent, especially in the treatment of **colorectal** and **breast cancer**. It is a **prodrug** that is enzymatically converted to **5-fluorouracil (5-FU)** in tumour cells, which allows for **selective targeting** of cancer cells while minimizing systemic toxicity. The inhibition of **thymidylate synthase** by 5-FU is critical for preventing the synthesis of thymidine, which is necessary for DNA replication. This mechanism disrupts cancer cell division, especially in rapidly proliferating cells.

Capecitabine's **oral administration** makes it more convenient compared to intravenous 5-FU, and it has been shown to be effective in various solid tumours. However, side effects such as **hand-foot syndrome**, **diarrhoea**, and **mucositis** must be monitored during treatment [1][2].

**Correct Answer: A) Inhibits thymidylate synthase resulting in impaired DNA synthesis**

## References

1. Van Cutsem E, Hoff PM, Harper P, et al. Oral capecitabine vs intravenous 5-fluorouracil and leucovorin: integrated analysis of two large, randomized, phase III trials in patients

with metastatic colorectal cancer. Ann Oncol. 2004;15(6):913-919.

2. Walko CM, Lindley C. Capecitabine: a review. Clin Ther. 2005;27(1):23-44.

---

*Table 6: Category of Chemotherapy*

| Category | Mechanism | Examples | Side Effects | Types |
|---|---|---|---|---|
| **Anti-Metabolites** | Inhibit DNA synthesis | Methotrexate, 5-FU, Fludarabine | Nausea, Myelosuppression, Mucositis, Alopecia | Purine Antagonists, Pyrimidine Antagonists |
| | | | Hand-foot syndrome, Diarrhoea, Liver damage | |
| **Vinca Alkaloids** | Prevent microtubule assembly | Vinblastine, Vincristine | Peripheral neuropathy, Myelosuppression | |
| | | | Loss of reflexes, Neurotoxicity | |
| **Alkylating Agents** | Cross-link DNA, preventing DNA repair | Cyclophosphamide, Ifosfamide | Haemorrhagic cystitis, Myelosuppression, Nausea | Nitrosoureas, Nitrogen Mustards |
| | | | Cardiotoxicity, Gonadotoxicity | |

| | | | | |
|---|---|---|---|---|
| **Platinum -based Agents** | Cross-link DNA, causing cell death | Cisplatin, Carboplatin, Oxaliplatin | Nephrotoxicity, Ototoxicity, Neurotoxicity | |
| | | | Myelosuppression | |
| **Taxanes** | Disrupt microtubule function | Docetaxel, Paclitaxel | Myelosuppression, Peripheral neuropathy | |
| | | | Myalgia, Arthralgia, Hypersensitivity reactions | |
| **Topoisomerase Inhibitors** | Prevent DNA unwinding during replication | Etoposide, Irinotecan | Alopecia, Myelosuppression, Diarrhea | Type I (Topoisomerase I Inhibitors), Type II (Topoisomerase II Inhibitors) |

## Case 91: Allopurinol and Azathioprine Interaction

### Clinical Scenario

A 58-year-old man is being treated with **azathioprine** for his autoimmune condition. His doctor decides to start him on **allopurinol** to prevent gout attacks. The doctor explains that careful monitoring is required due to a potential interaction between the two medications.

### Question

Which drug inhibits **xanthine oxidase** and requires caution when used with **azathioprine**?

A) Methotrexate
B) Cyclophosphamide
C) Allopurinol
D) 5-Fluorouracil
E) Dexamethasone

**Explanation**

**Allopurinol** is a **xanthine oxidase inhibitor. Azathioprine** is metabolized via **xanthine oxidase** into its active form, **6-mercaptopurine**. When allopurinol is used in conjunction with azathioprine, it inhibits the metabolism of azathioprine, leading to increased levels of **6-mercaptopurine** and a heightened risk of **toxicity**, particularly **myelosuppression**. Therefore, dose adjustment or close monitoring is required when both drugs are used together.

- **Option C** is correct: **Allopurinol** inhibits **xanthine oxidase**, necessitating caution when combined with azathioprine.

- **Option A** (Methotrexate) and **Option B** (Cyclophosphamide) are not metabolized by xanthine oxidase.

- **Option D** (5-Fluorouracil) and **Option E** (Dexamethasone) do not inhibit xanthine oxidase and are not related to this interaction.

**Advanced Surgical Talk**

**Allopurinol** is commonly used to treat **gout** and hyperuricemia by inhibiting **xanthine oxidase**, the enzyme responsible for converting hypoxanthine and xanthine into uric acid. However, because azathioprine is metabolized by the same enzyme pathway, concurrent use of allopurinol can lead to dangerously high levels of azathioprine's active metabolites, increasing the risk of **bone marrow suppression** and other toxicities.

Patients on both drugs should have their azathioprine dose reduced (typically by 50-75%) and should be monitored for signs of **myelosuppression**, including regular blood counts. This drug interaction is well-recognized and requires careful clinical management [1][2].

Correct Answer: C) Allopurinol

**References**

1.  Roberts RL, Barclay ML. Pharmacogenetics of azathioprine and 6-mercaptopurine metabolism and thiopurine S-methyltransferase deficiency. Pharmacogenetics. 2000;10(5):383-389.

2.  Relling MV, Schwab M, Whirl-Carrillo M, et al. Clinical pharmacogenetics implementation consortium guidelines for thiopurine methyltransferase genotype and thiopurine dosing: 2013 update. Clin Pharmacol Ther. 2013;93(4):324-325.

---

## Case 92: Mechanism of Action of Irinotecan

### Clinical Scenario

A 60-year-old woman with metastatic colorectal cancer is receiving chemotherapy with the **FOLFIRI** regimen, which includes **folinic acid**, **fluorouracil**, and **irinotecan**. The oncologist explains that irinotecan targets a specific phase of the cell cycle by inhibiting an important enzyme necessary for DNA replication.

### Question

Which drug in the **FOLFIRI** regimen is a **G2 phase inhibitor** that targets **topoisomerase I**?

A) Folinic acid
B) Fluorouracil
C) Irinotecan
D) Oxaliplatin
E) Leucovorin

### Explanation

**Irinotecan** is a **G2 phase inhibitor** and works by inhibiting **topoisomerase I**, an enzyme that facilitates the unwinding of DNA during replication. By inhibiting topoisomerase I, irinotecan prevents DNA from properly replicating, leading to DNA damage and apoptosis in cancer cells. It is a key component of the **FOLFIRI** regimen, which is commonly used in the treatment of **metastatic colorectal cancer**.

- **Option C is correct:** **Irinotecan** is a **G2 phase** inhibitor that targets **topoisomerase I**.

- **Option A** (Folinic acid) and **Option E** (Leucovorin) are used to enhance the effects of fluorouracil but do not inhibit topoisomerase.

- **Option B** (Fluorouracil) works by inhibiting thymidylate synthase, not topoisomerase.

- **Option D** (Oxaliplatin) is a platinum-based chemotherapy agent and works by cross-linking DNA, not by inhibiting topoisomerase.

## Advanced Surgical Talk

**Irinotecan** is a **topoisomerase I inhibitor** used primarily in the treatment of **colorectal cancer** as part of the **FOLFIRI** regimen. By inhibiting **topoisomerase I**, irinotecan disrupts DNA replication during the **G2 phase**, leading to DNA strand breaks and cell death. It is especially effective in rapidly dividing cancer cells where DNA replication is frequent.

The **FOLFIRI regimen** consists of:

- **Folinic acid** (leucovorin), which enhances the efficacy of fluorouracil,

- **Fluorouracil (5-FU)**, which inhibits thymidylate synthase, and

- **Irinotecan**, which inhibits topoisomerase I.

Common side effects of irinotecan include **diarrhoea**, **myelosuppression**, and **alopecia**, all of which require careful management during therapy [1][2].

**Correct Answer: C) Irinotecan**

## References

1. Pommier Y. Topoisomerase I inhibitors: camptothecins and beyond. Nat Rev Cancer. 2006;6(10):789-802.

2. Saltz LB, Cox JV, Blanke C, et al. Irinotecan plus fluorouracil and leucovorin for metastatic colorectal cancer. N Engl J Med. 2000;343(13):905-914.

*Table 7: chemotherapy regimens based on their cancer type*

| Category | Regimen | Drugs Included |
| --- | --- | --- |
| **Breast** | AC | Adriamycin (Doxorubicin), Cyclophosphamide |
| | CAF | Cyclophosphamide, Adriamycin (Doxorubicin), Fluorouracil (5-FU) |
| | CMF | Cyclophosphamide, Methotrexate, Fluorouracil (5-FU) |
| | CT | Cyclophosphamide, Taxotere (Docetaxel) |
| | EC | Epirubicin, Cyclophosphamide |
| | ECF | Epirubicin, Cisplatin, Fluorouracil (5-FU) |
| | FEC | Fluorouracil (5-FU), Epirubicin, Cyclophosphamide |
| | MMM | Methotrexate, Mitoxantrone, Mitomycin |
| **Colorectal** | FL (Mayo) | Fluorouracil (5-FU), Leucovorin (Folinic Acid) |
| | FOLFIRI | Fluorouracil (5-FU), Leucovorin (Folinic Acid), Irinotecan |
| | FOLFOX | Fluorouracil (5-FU), Leucovorin (Folinic Acid), Oxaliplatin |
| | FOLFOXIRI | Fluorouracil (5-FU), Leucovorin (Folinic Acid), Irinotecan, Oxaliplatin |
| **Pancreatic** | FOLFIRINOX | Fluorouracil (5-FU), Leucovorin (Folinic Acid), Irinotecan, Oxaliplatin |

| | Gemcitabine | Gemcitabine |
| --- | --- | --- |
| | GemCap | Gemcitabine, Capecitabine |
| **Gastro-Oesophageal** | ECF | Epirubicin, Cisplatin, Fluorouracil (5-FU) |
| | EOX | Epirubicin, Oxaliplatin, Capecitabine |
| | FAM | Fluorouracil (5-FU), Adriamycin (Doxorubicin), Mitomycin |
| | FAMTX | Fluorouracil (5-FU), Adriamycin (Doxorubicin), Mitomycin, Methotrexate |
| | FLOT | Fluorouracil (5-FU), Leucovorin (Folinic Acid), Oxaliplatin, Docetaxel |
| **Liver** | GemCap | Gemcitabine, Capecitabine |
| | GEMOX | Gemcitabine, Oxaliplatin |
| | MMM | Mitomycin, Methotrexate, Mitoxantrone |
| | TACE | Doxorubicin, Cisplatin |

## Case 93: Post-Renal Transplant Hernia Repair

### Clinical Scenario

A 55-year-old man presents with a **right iliac fossa mass** following a renal transplant several years ago. The mass has been slowly increasing in size, but the patient has no pain or other concerning symptoms. The surgical team discusses the possibility of a **hernia repair** and reviews the relevant guidelines.

### Question

What is the recommended approach for **hernia repair** in a patient with a history of renal transplant, according to the British Hernia Guidelines (2013)?

A) Laparoscopic repair is always recommended
B) Open repair is recommended due to the location of the

transplanted kidney
C) Laparoscopic repair is contraindicated
D) CT scan should always be performed to rule out occult malignancy
E) No intervention is needed unless symptomatic

**Explanation**

In this case, the **right iliac fossa mass** is most likely the **transplanted kidney**, which is commonly placed in the **pre-peritoneal space**. Hernias can occur in renal transplant patients due to the dissection involved in the transplant. The **British Hernia Guidelines (2013)** recommend **open repair** in such cases due to the technical challenges of laparoscopic repair in the presence of a transplanted kidney. While **laparoscopic repair** is feasible in experienced hands, **open repair** is the standard recommendation for this patient population.

- **Option B** is correct: The British Hernia Guidelines recommend **open repair** due to the anatomical location of the transplanted kidney.

- **Option A** (Laparoscopic repair is always recommended) is incorrect: Laparoscopic repair is possible but technically challenging in renal transplant patients.

- **Option C** (Laparoscopic repair is contraindicated) is incorrect because it may be feasible in experienced hands, but not routinely recommended.

- **Option D** (CT scan to rule out malignancy) may be useful if red flags are present, but in this case, it is unnecessary if the mass is clearly identified as the transplanted kidney.

- **Option E** (No intervention unless symptomatic) is incorrect, as hernias in renal transplant patients should be monitored and repaired as appropriate to avoid complications.

**Advanced Surgical Talk**

**Hernias** are relatively common in patients who have undergone **renal transplantation**, especially in the **right iliac fossa**, where the transplanted kidney is placed. The kidney is typically positioned in the **pre-peritoneal space**, which makes laparoscopic surgery more challenging due to the risk of damaging the transplanted organ or its vascular supply.

The **British Hernia Guidelines (2013)** suggest that **open repair** is generally safer in these patients. This approach allows for better control of the dissection and avoids the potential risks associated with the use of pneumoperitoneum during laparoscopic procedures. However, **laparoscopic repair** can be considered by highly experienced surgeons familiar with renal transplant anatomy. If there are no red flags (such as weight loss, night sweats, or unexplained pain), imaging is typically unnecessary unless malignancy or other pathology is suspected [1][2].

**Correct Answer: B) Open repair is recommended due to the location of the transplanted kidney**

### References

1.  Kingsnorth A, LeBlanc K. Hernias: inguinal and incisional. Lancet. 2003;362(9395):1561-1571.

2.  HerniaSurge Group. International guidelines for groin hernia management. Hernia. 2018;22(1):1-165.

## Case 94: Investigating Equivocal Hernia Symptoms

### Clinical Scenario

A 48-year-old man presents with intermittent **groin pain** and a mild bulge in the area, but physical examination is inconclusive for a hernia. The surgical team considers further imaging to clarify the diagnosis and refers to the European Hernia Society guidelines for appropriate investigation.

### Question

What is the **first-line** imaging modality recommended by the **European Hernia Society guidelines** for patients with **equivocal hernia symptoms**?

A) CT scan
B) MRI
C) Ultrasound (USS)
D) Laparoscopy
E) No further investigation unless symptoms worsen

### Explanation

The **European Hernia Society guidelines** recommend **ultrasound (USS)** as the **first-line investigation** for patients with **equivocal hernia symptoms**. Ultrasound is non-invasive, widely available, and provides a good assessment of soft tissue structures in the groin area, making it the preferred initial investigation for identifying hernias when physical examination findings are unclear.

If the **ultrasound** results are inconclusive, further imaging with **CT** or **MRI** can be considered. These modalities provide more detailed cross-sectional imaging and are useful in complex or unclear cases, but they are not typically the first choice due to their cost and accessibility.

- **Option C** is correct: **Ultrasound (USS)** is the recommended first-line imaging modality for equivocal hernia symptoms.

- **Option A** (CT scan) and **Option B** (MRI) are second-line investigations, used when ultrasound results are inconclusive.

- **Option D** (Laparoscopy) is not indicated for diagnosis; it is used primarily for hernia repair.

- **Option E** (No further investigation unless symptoms worsen) is incorrect, as ultrasound is recommended in equivocal cases.

## Advanced Surgical Talk

In cases where **hernia symptoms** are equivocal or **physical examination** is inconclusive, the **European Hernia Society guidelines** recommend **ultrasound** as the **first-line investigation**. Ultrasound is effective in identifying various types of hernias, including **inguinal, femoral**, and **spigelian** hernias, and it provides dynamic assessment, such as identifying herniation during straining.

If the ultrasound does not yield clear results or if there is suspicion of a more complex hernia (such as an **incarcerated hernia** or one involving other abdominal organs), a **CT** or **MRI** scan can be employed. These imaging modalities offer more detailed views and are useful in cases of **recurrent hernias**, previous surgery, or unclear anatomy.

Ultrasound remains the **go-to** diagnostic tool due to its availability, cost-effectiveness, and ability to provide real-time imaging in various clinical settings [1][2].

**Correct Answer: C) Ultrasound (USS)**

**References**

1. Simons MP, Aufenacker T, Bay-Nielsen M, et al. European Hernia Society guidelines on the treatment of inguinal hernia in adult patients. Hernia. 2009;13(4):343-403.

2. Robinson A, Light D, Nice C. Groin hernias: current thought on diagnosis and management. Surgeon. 2015;13(4):195-202.

## Case 95: European Hernia Guidelines

### Clinical Scenario

A 62-year-old man presents with a **large inguinal hernia** that appears to extend into the **scrotum**. The surgical team discusses the key factors outlined in the **European Hernia Society guidelines** that should be considered when planning the surgical approach.

### Question

Which factor is **not** included as a specific component in the **European Hernia Society guidelines** for hernia classification?

A) Size of hernia defect
B) Scrotal involvement
C) Duration of hernia
D) Symptoms of pain or discomfort
E) Previous hernia surgery

### Explanation

The **European Hernia Society guidelines** include several key components for the classification and management of **inguinal hernias**, such as the **size of the hernia defect, duration of the hernia, symptoms**, and whether the patient has had **previous hernia surgery**. However, **scrotal involvement** is **not** specifically listed as a primary classification criterion in the guidelines.

While **scrotal involvement** may influence the complexity of the hernia repair, it is not considered a core component of the classification system outlined in the European Hernia guidelines. The other listed components are directly related to the decision-making process for surgical management.

- **Option B** is correct: **Scrotal involvement** is not a specific classification component in the **European Hernia Society guidelines**.

- **Option A** (Size of hernia defect) is part of the classification system, influencing the type of repair needed.

- **Option C** (Duration of hernia) is relevant to determining the likelihood of complications or recurrence.

- **Option D** (Symptoms of pain or discomfort) is important for determining the need for surgical intervention.

- **Option E** (Previous hernia surgery) is a significant factor in planning the surgical approach.

**Advanced Surgical Talk**

The **European Hernia Society guidelines** provide a framework for classifying and managing **inguinal hernias** based on factors such as the **size of the hernia defect**, the **duration of symptoms**, the presence of **pain or discomfort**, and whether the patient has had any **previous hernia repairs**. These factors help guide the choice between **open** and **laparoscopic** approaches, as well as the type of mesh used.

While **scrotal involvement** can complicate hernia repair, particularly in cases of **scrotal hernias** (hernia extending into the scrotum), it is not specifically listed as a core component of the guidelines. Nonetheless, scrotal hernias may require more complex repairs, especially if there is **testicular involvement** or other anatomical challenges. In these cases, an **open repair** may be preferred, although experienced surgeons may still opt for a **laparoscopic approach** in some cases [1][2].

**Correct Answer: B) Scrotal involvement**

**References**


1.  Simons MP, Aufenacker T, Bay-Nielsen M, et al. European Hernia Society guidelines on the treatment of inguinal hernia in adult patients. Hernia. 2009;13(4):343-403.

2.  Miserez M, Peeters E, Aufenacker T, et al. The European Hernia Society groin hernia classification: simple and easy to remember. Hernia. 2007;11(2):113-116.

# Case 96: Hernia Repair in Patients Preferring No Mesh

## Clinical Scenario

A 50-year-old man with a **right inguinal hernia** expresses concern about the use of mesh in his hernia repair. After discussing his options with the surgical team, the patient is still hesitant about mesh and asks for alternative approaches.

## Question

According to the **European Hernia Society guidelines**, what is the recommended hernia repair technique for patients who prefer not to use mesh?

A) Lichtenstein repair
B) Laparoscopic repair
C) Shouldice repair
D) TAPP repair
E) Watchful waiting

## Explanation

The **European Hernia Society guidelines** emphasize that, when possible, a **mesh repair** should be recommended for inguinal hernias due to its lower recurrence rate. However, in patients who **refuse mesh**, the guidelines recommend the **Shouldice repair** as the alternative. The **Shouldice repair** is a **tissue-based** repair technique that uses multiple layers of the patient's own tissues to reinforce the inguinal canal without mesh. This technique is associated with relatively low recurrence rates when performed by experienced surgeons.

- **Option C** is correct: The **Shouldice repair** is recommended for patients who refuse mesh in hernia repair.

- **Option A** (Lichtenstein repair) involves the use of mesh, which the patient has declined.

- **Option B** (Laparoscopic repair) typically involves mesh as well.

- **Option D** (TAPP repair) is a laparoscopic approach that also uses mesh.

- **Option E** (Watchful waiting) may be an option in asymptomatic patients, but it is not a repair technique.

**Advanced Surgical Talk**

The **Shouldice repair** is a well-established, non-mesh, tissue-based repair for **inguinal hernias**. It involves meticulous dissection and suturing of **four layers** of the inguinal canal. This method is known for its low recurrence rate when performed at specialized centres, though it requires more surgical skill and time compared to mesh-based repairs.

The **European Hernia Society guidelines** highlight the importance of a **shared decision-making process** between the patient and the surgeon. If a patient strongly prefers not to have a **mesh repair**, the Shouldice technique is considered the best alternative. Although mesh-based repairs (such as **Lichtenstein** and **laparoscopic** approaches) are associated with lower recurrence rates overall, the Shouldice repair remains a viable option, particularly for patients with concerns about foreign materials [1][2].

**Correct Answer: C) Shouldice repair**

**References**


1. Simons MP, Aufenacker T, Bay-Nielsen M, et al. European Hernia Society guidelines on the treatment of inguinal hernia in adult patients. Hernia. 2009;13(4):343-403.

2. Kingsnorth A, LeBlanc K. Hernias: inguinal and incisional. Lancet. 2003;362(9395):1561-1571.


---

## Case 97: Mesh and Non-Mesh Hernia Repair Options

**Clinical Scenario**

A 45-year-old man with a **left inguinal hernia** is scheduled for surgery. He is informed about various types of **hernia repair techniques**, including mesh and non-mesh options. The surgical team discusses different repair methods and explains that the **European Hernia Society (EHS)** recommends the **Shouldice repair** as the best non-mesh option.

**Question**

Which of the following is a **mesh repair** technique placed in the **preperitoneal space**?

A) Bassini repair
B) Shouldice repair

C) Desarda repair
D) McVay repair
E) Kugel repair

**Explanation**

The **Kugel repair** is a **mesh-based** repair technique where the mesh is placed in the **preperitoneal space** to cover the hernia defect. This allows for a tension-free repair with low recurrence rates. The **preperitoneal space** is the area between the peritoneum and the transversalis fascia, and placing the mesh here provides robust support without entering the abdominal cavity.

The **Bassini, Shouldice**, and **Desarda** repairs are all **non-mesh** techniques that use suturing of the patient's tissues to reinforce the inguinal canal. Among these, the **Shouldice repair** is the most widely recommended non-mesh option by the **European Hernia Society (EHS)**.

- **Option E** is correct: The **Kugel repair** is a **mesh repair** placed in the **preperitoneal space**.

- **Option A** (Bassini repair) and **Option B** (Shouldice repair) are non-mesh repairs.

- **Option C** (Desarda repair) is also a non-mesh tissue-based repair.

- **Option D** (McVay repair) is another non-mesh technique used for hernia repairs.

**Advanced Surgical Talk**

The **Kugel repair** is a unique **mesh-based technique** that involves placing the mesh in the **preperitoneal space** through a small incision, allowing for a tension-free hernia repair. It is particularly useful for **inguinal** and **ventral hernias** and provides strong reinforcement of the abdominal wall.

In contrast, non-mesh techniques like the **Shouldice** and **Bassini** repairs rely on suturing the patient's tissues, which can result in higher tension and potentially higher recurrence rates compared to mesh repairs. However, in certain patients who are uncomfortable with mesh implants or have specific contraindications, the **Shouldice repair** is often recommended by the **European Hernia Society (EHS)** as the best non-mesh option due to its low recurrence rate when performed correctly [1][2].

**Correct Answer: E) Kugel repair**

## References

1.  Simons MP, Aufenacker T, Bay-Nielsen M, et al. European Hernia Society guidelines on the treatment of inguinal hernia in adult patients. Hernia. 2009;13(4):343-403.

2.  Kingsnorth A, LeBlanc K. Hernias: inguinal and incisional. Lancet. 2003;362(9395):1561-1571.

## Case 98: Use of Antibiotics in Hernia Repair

### Clinical Scenario

A 60-year-old man with a **recurrent inguinal hernia** is scheduled for **laparoscopic hernia repair**. The surgical team discusses whether antibiotics are needed before the procedure, as the patient is concerned about infection.

### Question

According to the **European Hernia Society guidelines**, what is the recommendation regarding the use of antibiotics in **laparoscopic hernia repair**?

A) Antibiotics should always be used
B) Antibiotics are recommended only for recurrent hernias
C) Antibiotics are recommended for laparoscopic repairs
D) Antibiotics are generally not recommended for laparoscopic repairs
E) Antibiotics are mandatory for all hernia surgeries

### Explanation

The **European Hernia Society guidelines** state that **antibiotics are generally not recommended** for **laparoscopic hernia repairs** due to the low risk of infection associated with these procedures. **Laparoscopic hernia repair** is a minimally invasive surgery, and the incidence of wound infections is significantly lower compared to open repairs.

In contrast, for **open hernia repairs**, antibiotics may be considered if there is concern about infection (e.g., in high-risk patients or cases involving large, complex hernias), but they are not routinely required.

- **Option D** is correct: **Antibiotics are generally not recommended** for **laparoscopic hernia repairs**.

- **Option A** (antibiotics should always be used) is incorrect because antibiotics are not routinely recommended for laparoscopic repairs.

- **Option B** is incorrect because the need for antibiotics is not determined solely by whether the hernia is recurrent.

- **Option C** (antibiotics are recommended for laparoscopic repairs) is incorrect, as they are generally not recommended.

- **Option E** (antibiotics are mandatory for all hernia surgeries) is incorrect, as the use of antibiotics is not required for all hernia surgeries.

**Advanced Surgical Talk**

The **European Hernia Society** has clear guidelines regarding the use of **prophylactic antibiotics** in hernia surgery. For **laparoscopic inguinal hernia repairs**, the risk of surgical site infection is low, and therefore routine administration of antibiotics is not necessary. This is due to the smaller incisions, reduced exposure of tissues, and lower overall infection risk compared to open procedures.

However, in certain circumstances, such as **open hernia repairs** or patients with **high risk factors** (e.g., obesity, diabetes, immunosuppression), antibiotics may be considered to reduce the risk of infection. Surgeons should assess the patient's individual risk factors before deciding whether antibiotics are needed in cases where infection risk is a concern [1][2].

Correct Answer: D) Antibiotics are generally not recommended for laparoscopic repairs

**References**

1. Simons MP, Aufenacker T, Bay-Nielsen M, et al. European Hernia Society guidelines on the treatment of inguinal hernia in adult patients. Hernia. 2009;13(4):343-403.

2. Aufenacker TJ, Koelemay MJ, Gouma DJ, Simons MP. Systematic review and meta-analysis of the effectiveness of antibiotic prophylaxis in prevention of wound infection after mesh repair of abdominal wall hernia. Br J Surg. 2006;93(1):5-10.

## Clinical Scenario

A 65-year-old man with a **colostomy** following a previous surgery for rectal cancer is concerned about the risk of developing a **parastomal hernia**. The surgical team discusses the risk factors and incidence of parastomal hernia in patients with stomas, as outlined by the European Hernia Society (EHS).

## Question

According to the **European Hernia Society (EHS)**, what percentage of patients with a stoma will develop a **parastomal hernia** within the first 12 months?

A) 10%
B) 15%
C) 30%
D) 50%
E) 70%

## Explanation

The **European Hernia Society (EHS)** estimates that approximately **30%** of all patients with a stoma will develop a **parastomal hernia** within the first **12 months**. This risk is particularly high in patients with an **end colostomy** and increases with the **duration** of time the patient has the stoma.

- **Option C** is correct: Around **30%** of patients with a stoma will develop a **parastomal hernia** within 12 months.

- **Option A** (10%) and **Option B** (15%) underestimate the risk.

- **Option D** (50%) and **Option E** (70%) overestimate the incidence of parastomal hernia within the first year.

## Advanced Surgical Talk

A **parastomal hernia** is a common complication in patients with a stoma. The risk of developing a parastomal hernia is higher in patients with an **end colostomy** compared to those with a loop colostomy or ileostomy. The risk also increases over time, with the highest incidence typically seen within the first year after stoma creation.

Other risk factors for parastomal hernia development include **obesity, chronic cough, physical strain**, and **poor wound**

**healing**. The EHS guidelines recommend that patients with a stoma be regularly monitored for hernia development, and preventive measures, such as **stoma support belts** or **surgical mesh reinforcement**, may be considered for high-risk patients [1][2].

**Correct Answer: C) 30%**

## References


1. Lambrecht JR, Eikrem ØS, Øresland T. Parastomal hernias and indications for repair. Scand J Surg. 2013;102(2):62-66.

2. Antoniou SA, Agresta F, Garcia Alamino JM, et al. European Hernia Society guidelines on prevention and treatment of parastomal hernias. Hernia. 2018;22(1):183-198.


## Case 100: Prophylactic Mesh for Parastomal Hernia

### Clinical Scenario

A 60-year-old woman is scheduled for an **end colostomy** as part of her treatment for rectal cancer. During the preoperative consultation, the surgeon discusses the potential for developing a **parastomal hernia** and the option of using **prophylactic mesh** during the stoma creation to reduce this risk.

### Question

What is the current evidence regarding the use of **prophylactic mesh** for reducing the risk of **parastomal hernia** in patients undergoing stoma formation?

A) Prophylactic mesh is proven to significantly reduce parastomal hernia rates
B) Prophylactic mesh has no effect on parastomal hernia rates
C) The Stoma-Const trial showed no significant difference in hernia rates with or without mesh
D) Prophylactic mesh is not recommended due to high complication rates
E) CT-based diagnosis of hernias suggests that mesh increases hernia incidence

### Explanation

There is evidence supporting the use of **prophylactic mesh** in reducing the risk of **parastomal hernia**, particularly in patients with **permanent stomas**. However, the **Stoma-Const trial** found **no significant difference** in hernia rates between patients with and without prophylactic mesh. It is important to note that the trial used **CT scans** to diagnose hernias, which may **overestimate** the incidence of parastomal hernias due to its high sensitivity.

Additionally, there may have been **heterogeneity** in the types of stoma formations used in the study, which could have influenced the outcomes. Despite the trial's findings, many surgeons still advocate for the use of prophylactic mesh, especially in cases where a **permanent stoma** is planned, as it intuitively makes sense to reinforce the area at the time of surgery.

- **Option C** is correct: The **Stoma-Const trial** showed no significant difference in hernia rates with or without mesh.

- **Option A** (proven to reduce hernia rates) is incorrect, as the trial did not show a significant reduction.

- **Option B** (no effect) oversimplifies the nuanced findings, as there is conflicting evidence in the literature.

- **Option D** (not recommended due to complications) is incorrect, as prophylactic mesh is not associated with high complication rates in this context.

- **Option E** (increases hernia incidence) is incorrect; the **CT-based** diagnosis may overestimate the hernia incidence, but mesh does not increase the risk of hernias.

**Advanced Surgical Talk**

**Prophylactic mesh placement** has been debated as a strategy to prevent **parastomal hernias**, which are a common complication of stoma creation. Some studies suggest that mesh can reduce hernia rates, particularly when used in **permanent stomas** like end colostomies. However, the **Stoma-Const trial** introduced doubt by showing **no significant reduction** in hernia rates, though the use of **CT scans** for diagnosis might have influenced the results by overestimating the true incidence.

The decision to use **prophylactic mesh** should be individualized based on patient factors, the type of stoma, and the surgeon's experience. While some centres routinely use mesh for permanent stomas, others may reserve it for high-risk patients, such as those with **obesity** or previous abdominal surgery [1][2].

Correct Answer: C) The Stoma-Const trial showed no significant difference in hernia rates with or without mesh

**References**

1. Hansson BM, Helgstrand F, Jorgensen LN, et al. Prophylactic mesh placement for the prevention of parastomal hernia: a systematic review and meta-analysis. Ann Surg. 2012;255(4):707-714.

2. Hauters P, Cardin JL, Lepere M, et al. Prophylactic mesh does not prevent parastomal hernia in end-colostomies: Stoma-Const trial results. Ann Surg. 2019;270(4):639-645.

## Case 101: Prophylactic Mesh in Stoma Creation

### Clinical Scenario

A 68-year-old man undergoing an **end colostomy** is concerned about developing a **parastomal hernia**. The surgical team discusses the option of using **prophylactic mesh** during the surgery to reduce the risk of hernia formation. The patient asks about the latest evidence on whether the use of mesh is effective in preventing parastomal hernias.

### Question

What is the best approach to potentially reduce the risk of **parastomal hernia** in a patient undergoing stoma formation, according to recent studies?

A) Mesh insertion
B) Laparoscopic stoma creation
C) Avoiding mesh due to higher complication rates
D) Reversing the stoma after a year
E) Using absorbable sutures for stoma creation

### Explanation

There is evidence suggesting that **prophylactic mesh** insertion during stoma creation can reduce the incidence of **parastomal hernias**, particularly in cases of **permanent stomas** such as **end colostomies**. However, the recent **Stoma-Const trial** found **no significant difference** in hernia rates between patients who received mesh and those who did not. The trial used **CT scans** as the primary diagnostic tool, which may have overestimated the incidence of parastomal hernias.

Despite these findings, many surgeons continue to advocate for **mesh placement**, particularly in cases where a **permanent stoma** is planned. Mesh can help reinforce the abdominal wall around the stoma site and potentially lower the risk of hernia formation, even if the most recent trial showed no definitive statistical difference.

- **Option A** is correct: **Mesh insertion** is still considered a potential strategy for reducing parastomal hernia rates, especially in patients with permanent stomas.

- **Option B** (laparoscopic stoma creation) does not specifically reduce parastomal hernia rates.

- **Option C** (avoiding mesh due to higher complication rates) is incorrect, as mesh has not been associated with significant complication rates in this context.

- **Option D** (reversing the stoma after a year) may not be feasible for many patients, particularly those requiring a permanent stoma.

- **Option E** (using absorbable sutures) is not supported by evidence as a method to prevent parastomal hernias.

## Advanced Surgical Talk

**Prophylactic mesh** is often placed during stoma creation to reduce the risk of **parastomal hernia**, a common complication in patients with stomas. While studies such as the **Stoma-Const trial** have raised questions about its efficacy, the use of mesh still makes **intuitive sense**, particularly for **permanent stomas**. Mesh provides structural support to the abdominal wall, decreasing the likelihood of herniation through the stoma site.

The **Stoma-Const trial** found **no statistically significant difference** between mesh and non-mesh groups, but it relied on **CT-based diagnosis**, which may have overestimated hernia rates. Additionally, heterogeneity in stoma types may have influenced the results. Despite this, mesh remains a viable option, especially for patients with risk factors such as **obesity**, **advanced age**, or those requiring a permanent stoma [1][2].

Correct Answer: A) Mesh insertion

## References

1. Hansson BM, Helgstrand F, Jorgensen LN, et al. Prophylactic mesh placement for the prevention of parastomal hernia: a systematic review and meta-analysis. Ann Surg. 2012;255(4):707-714.

2. Hauters P, Cardin JL, Lepere M, et al. Prophylactic mesh does not prevent parastomal hernia in end-colostomies: Stoma-Const trial results. Ann Surg. 2019;270(4):639-645.

## Case 102: Tranexamic Acid in Bleeding

### Clinical Scenario

A 72-year-old man is admitted with a **gastrointestinal bleed**. The surgical team is discussing the use of **tranexamic acid (TXA)** to reduce bleeding, but they refer to recent evidence, including the **HALT-IT trial**, which raises concerns about its efficacy and safety in this context.

### Question

What does recent evidence, including the **HALT-IT trial**, suggest about the use of **tranexamic acid (TXA)** in patients with **gastrointestinal bleeding**?

A) TXA reduces bleeding with no significant side effects
B) TXA is beneficial in trauma patients and gastrointestinal bleeds
C) TXA has no benefit in gastrointestinal bleeds and may increase thromboembolic events
D) TXA is recommended for gastrointestinal bleeds according to current guidelines
E) TXA is safe and effective for use in all types of bleeding

### Explanation

While **tranexamic acid (TXA)** has demonstrated benefits in **trauma patients** by reducing bleeding and improving outcomes, its role in **gastrointestinal (GI) bleeding** has been called into question. The **HALT-IT trial** found **no significant benefit** of TXA in reducing mortality or rebleeding in patients with GI bleeds. Furthermore, the trial raised concerns about a potential increase in **thromboembolic events** in patients who received TXA, suggesting that it may be harmful in this setting.

- **Option C is correct:** The **HALT-IT trial** suggests that TXA has **no benefit** in gastrointestinal bleeds and may increase the risk of thromboembolic events.

- **Option A is incorrect:** TXA has not been shown to reduce bleeding without significant risks in GI bleeds.

- **Option B** is incorrect: While TXA is beneficial in **trauma patients**, it is not beneficial in gastrointestinal bleeds.

- **Option D** is incorrect: Current guidelines do not recommend TXA for GI bleeds due to the findings of the HALT-IT trial.

- **Option E** is incorrect: TXA is not universally safe and effective for all types of bleeding, particularly gastrointestinal bleeds.

## Advanced Surgical Talk

**Tranexamic acid (TXA)** works by inhibiting fibrinolysis, helping to stabilize clots and reduce bleeding. While it has been beneficial in trauma settings, its use in **gastrointestinal bleeding** has not shown the same positive outcomes. The **HALT-IT trial** specifically investigated the use of TXA in patients with **upper and lower GI bleeding** and found **no reduction in mortality**, rebleeding, or the need for interventions like blood transfusions.

More concerning were the findings of increased rates of **venous thromboembolism** (VTE), including deep vein thrombosis and pulmonary embolism, in patients treated with TXA. Given these risks and the lack of benefit, the use of TXA in gastrointestinal bleeds is not currently recommended, and its role in these patients remains highly questionable [1][2].

**Correct Answer: C) TXA has no benefit in gastrointestinal bleeds and may increase thromboembolic events**

## References


1. Roberts I, Shakur-Still H, Afolabi A, et al. HALT-IT—tranexamic acid for the treatment of gastrointestinal bleeding: an international randomised, double-blind, placebo-controlled trial. Lancet. 2020;395(10241):1927-1936.

2. Hunt BJ. The current place of tranexamic acid in the management of bleeding. Anaesthesia. 2015;70(Suppl 1):50-53.

## Clinical Scenario

A 68-year-old man presents to the emergency department with **frank melena** (indicating gastrointestinal bleeding) and an oxygen saturation of **90%**. The emergency nurse asks about the immediate management steps.

## Question

Which of the following interventions would you **not** institute in this patient's initial management?

A) IV fluids
B) Tranexamic acid
C) Urinary catheter
D) Oxygen supplementation
E) Blood transfusion

## Explanation

The immediate management of a patient presenting with gastrointestinal bleeding (melena) and low oxygen saturation includes **IV fluids** to maintain blood pressure, **oxygen supplementation** to address hypoxia, and a **urinary catheter** to monitor urine output. If the patient is hemodynamically unstable or has significant anaemia, a **blood transfusion** may be indicated.

However, based on the **HALT-IT trial**, the use of **tranexamic acid** in gastrointestinal bleeding is **not recommended**. The study found that TXA did not reduce mortality or rebleeding rates and was associated with an increased risk of **thromboembolic events**.

- **Option B** is correct: **Tranexamic acid** is not recommended in the management of gastrointestinal bleeding.

- **Option A** (IV fluids) is appropriate to stabilize the patient.

- **Option C** (Urinary catheter) is useful for monitoring renal function and volume status.

- **Option D** (Oxygen supplementation) is necessary due to the patient's low oxygen saturation.

- **Option E** (Blood transfusion) may be considered based on the patient's haemoglobin levels and clinical status.

**Advanced Surgical Talk**

In the management of **acute gastrointestinal bleeding**, rapid stabilization of the patient is critical. This includes **IV fluid resuscitation**, **oxygen supplementation**, and monitoring with a **urinary catheter**. If there is significant blood loss, a **blood transfusion** should be considered. However, the use of **tranexamic acid** in GI bleeds has been shown to provide no significant benefit in reducing mortality or rebleeding, and it may increase the risk of thromboembolic complications [1][2].

**Correct Answer: B) Tranexamic acid**

**References**

1. Roberts I, Shakur-Still H, Afolabi A, et al. HALT-IT—tranexamic acid for the treatment of gastrointestinal bleeding: an international randomised, double-blind, placebo-controlled trial. Lancet. 2020;395(10241):1927-1936.

2. Gralnek IM, Dumonceau JM, Kuipers EJ, et al. Diagnosis and management of nonvariceal upper gastrointestinal hemorrhage: European Society of Gastrointestinal Endoscopy (ESGE) Guideline. Endoscopy. 2015;47(10).

## Case 105: Antibiotics Targeting the 30S Ribosome

**Clinical Scenario**

A 40-year-old woman is prescribed an antibiotic for her **urinary tract infection**. The doctor explains that the drug works by inhibiting the **30S ribosomal subunit**, preventing bacterial protein synthesis.

**Question**

Which antibiotic acts by inhibiting the **30S ribosomal subunit**?

A) Azithromycin
B) Tetracycline
C) Erythromycin
D) Clindamycin
E) Rifampicin

**Explanation**

Antibiotics that target the **30S ribosomal subunit** prevent bacterial protein synthesis, which leads to bacterial cell death or the inhibition of bacterial growth. **Tetracycline** is an antibiotic that binds to the **30S subunit** of bacterial ribosomes, thereby inhibiting protein synthesis.

- **Option B** is correct: **Tetracycline** acts by inhibiting the **30S ribosomal subunit**.

- **Option A** (Azithromycin) and **Option C** (Erythromycin) are **macrolide antibiotics** that act on the **50S ribosomal subunit**, not the 30S subunit.

- **Option D** (Clindamycin) also targets the **50S ribosomal subunit**, not the 30S subunit.

- **Option E** (Rifampicin) inhibits bacterial RNA polymerase, not the ribosome.

## Advanced Surgical Talk

Antibiotics that inhibit the **30S ribosomal subunit**, such as **tetracyclines** and **aminoglycosides**, are bacteriostatic or bactericidal agents that disrupt bacterial protein synthesis. **Tetracyclines** block the attachment of aminoacyl-tRNA to the ribosomal complex, preventing the addition of new amino acids to the growing peptide chain. This mechanism of action is particularly effective against a wide range of bacterial infections, including **urinary tract infections**, **acne**, and **chlamydia**.

In contrast, **macrolides** (such as **erythromycin** and **azithromycin**) target the **50S subunit**, and **rifampicin** acts on bacterial **RNA polymerase**. Understanding the specific targets of these antibiotics is essential for their appropriate clinical use and for avoiding resistance development [1][2].

**Correct Answer: B) Tetracycline**

## References


1. Chopra I, Roberts M. Tetracycline antibiotics: mode of action, applications, molecular biology, and epidemiology of bacterial resistance. Microbiol Mol Biol Rev. 2001;65(2):232-260.

2. Wilson DN. Ribosome-targeting antibiotics and mechanisms of bacterial resistance. Nat Rev Microbiol. 2014;12(1):35-48.

## Clinical Scenario

A 65-year-old woman is admitted with symptoms of a severe bacterial infection. Her blood work reveals elevated levels of **C-reactive protein (CRP)**, which prompts the medical team to discuss its origins and significance.

## Question

Why is **C-reactive protein (CRP)** termed with the letter **C**?

A) It reacts with a carbohydrate on the pneumococcal capsule
B) It was originally discovered in cholera patients
C) It was named after its discovery in cancer patients
D) It reacts with complement proteins in the immune system
E) It is related to coagulation factors in sepsis

## Explanation

**C-reactive protein (CRP)** was originally discovered in the context of **pneumonia** caused by **pneumococcus** bacteria. The "C" in CRP refers to its ability to bind to the **C-polysaccharide** (a component of the **capsule**) on the surface of **Streptococcus pneumoniae**. CRP is part of the **innate immune response** and is elevated in response to inflammation and infection.

- **Option A** is correct: The "C" in CRP comes from its reaction with the **C-polysaccharide** of the pneumococcal capsule.

- **Option B** (cholera) is incorrect, as CRP was not named after cholera.

- **Option C** (cancer) is incorrect, as CRP was discovered in the context of pneumococcal infection, not cancer.

- **Option D** (complement) is related to CRP's immune functions, but the name comes from its reactivity with the C-polysaccharide.

- **Option E** (coagulation) is incorrect, as CRP is not primarily related to coagulation factors.

## Advanced Surgical Talk

**C-reactive protein (CRP)** is an **acute-phase protein** that increases in response to inflammation, infection, and tissue injury. It was originally discovered in patients with **pneumococcal pneumonia**, where it was observed to react with the **C-**

**polysaccharide** of the pneumococcal capsule. This reaction led to its naming as **C-reactive protein**.

CRP plays a role in the **innate immune response** by binding to microbial polysaccharides and activating the **complement system**, which enhances phagocytosis and helps to eliminate pathogens. Elevated CRP levels are commonly used as a **biomarker** for systemic inflammation and infection, especially in conditions such as **sepsis, pneumonia**, and **autoimmune diseases** [1][2].

**Correct Answer: A) It reacts with a carbohydrate on the pneumococcal capsule**

### References


1. Volanakis JE. Human C-reactive protein: expression, structure, and function. Mol Immunol. 2001;38(2-3):189-197.

2. Black S, Kushner I, Samols D. C-reactive protein. J Biol Chem. 2004;279(47):48487-48490.


---

## Case 107: D-Dimer

### Clinical Scenario

A 70-year-old man is admitted with suspected **disseminated intravascular coagulation (DIC)** following sepsis. His lab results show elevated **D-dimer** levels, and the medical team discusses the significance of D-dimer values in diagnosing DIC.

### Question

Which of the following D-dimer levels is significant in diagnosing **disseminated intravascular coagulation (DIC)**?

A) D-dimer of 10 mg/L
B) D-dimer of 100 µg/L
C) D-dimer of 100 ng/mL
D) D-dimer of 500 µg/L
E) D-dimer of 1000 ng/L

### Explanation

In the context of **disseminated intravascular coagulation (DIC)**, **D-dimer** is commonly elevated due to increased fibrin degradation. D-dimer levels are typically reported in **ng/mL** or **µg/L**, with higher levels indicating a greater degree of clot breakdown. A D-dimer level of **1000 ng/L** is commonly used as a threshold for concern in cases of DIC. It is important to note the **difference in units** when interpreting D-dimer values, as D-dimer may be reported in different measurement systems.

- **Option E** is correct: A **D-dimer level of 1000 ng/L** is significant in diagnosing DIC.

- **Option A** (10 mg/L) is very high but unlikely to be a standard reporting unit for D-dimer.

- **Option B** (100 µg/L) and **Option D** (500 µg/L) are lower but not as commonly used in DIC diagnosis.

- **Option C** (100 ng/mL) is significant but lower than the threshold for concern in DIC.

**Advanced Surgical Talk**

**D-dimer** is a product of fibrin degradation and is used as a marker for **coagulation activity**. In **disseminated intravascular coagulation (DIC)**, the body experiences excessive clot formation followed by widespread clot breakdown, leading to elevated D-dimer levels. It is important to recognize the **units** in which D-dimer is reported. Typically, D-dimer levels are significant when above **500 ng/mL** (or **1000 ng/L**), depending on the lab's reporting standards.

In DIC, D-dimer is used along with other tests (e.g., **platelet count**, **fibrinogen levels**, **prothrombin time**) to assess the degree of coagulation dysfunction. Elevated D-dimer levels in DIC indicate ongoing clot breakdown, which is a hallmark of the disorder [1][2].

Correct Answer: E) D-dimer of 1000 ng/L

**References**


1. Taylor FB Jr, Toh CH, Hoots WK, et al. Towards definition, clinical and laboratory criteria, and a scoring system for disseminated intravascular coagulation: on behalf of the Scientific Subcommittee on Disseminated Intravascular Coagulation (DIC) of the International Society on Thrombosis and Haemostasis (ISTH). Thromb Haemost. 2001;86(5):1327-1330.

2. Levi M, Ten Cate H. Disseminated intravascular coagulation. N Engl J Med. 1999;341(8):586-592.

## Clinical Scenario

A 52-year-old man presents with a visible **umbilical hernia**. On physical examination, the hernia is clearly apparent, and the surgical team discusses whether any additional imaging is necessary to confirm the diagnosis.

## Question

According to the **European Hernia Society (EHS)** and **American Hernia Society (AHS)** guidelines, what imaging is required when the diagnosis of **umbilical hernia** is clearly visible on physical examination?

A) CT scan
B) Ultrasound (USS)
C) Dynamic ultrasound
D) MRI
E) None required

## Explanation

According to the **EHS** and **AHS guidelines**, when a **hernia** is **clearly visible** on physical examination, no additional imaging is necessary to confirm the diagnosis. If the hernia is palpable and easily identified, further imaging would not alter the management plan, and unnecessary imaging can be avoided.

- **Option E** is correct: If the hernia is clearly visible on physical examination, **no imaging** is required.

- **Option A** (CT scan), **Option B** (Ultrasound), **Option C** (Dynamic ultrasound), and **Option D** (MRI) are not indicated when the hernia is clearly present.

## Advanced Surgical Talk

In cases of **umbilical hernia**, clinical examination is usually sufficient to make the diagnosis if the hernia is clearly visible. The **European Hernia Society (EHS)** and **American Hernia Society (AHS)** guidelines recommend that imaging studies (such as **CT scans**, **ultrasounds**, or **MRIs**) are only necessary in cases where the hernia is not easily identifiable, or if the patient has **equivocal symptoms**.

For more complex or **recurrent hernias**, or when the diagnosis is uncertain, imaging modalities like **CT** or **dynamic ultrasound** can be used to assess the hernia's size, contents, and whether there is any

**incarceration** or **strangulation**. However, in the case of a clearly visible hernia, imaging is not required, and the focus should shift to planning the **surgical repair** if indicated [1][2].



### References


1. Muysoms FE, Miserez M, Berrevoet F, et al. Classification of primary and incisional abdominal wall hernias. Hernia. 2009;13(4):407-414.

2. Awad SS, Fagan SP. Current approaches to inguinal hernia repair. Am J Surg. 2004;188(6A Suppl):9S-16S.


## Case 109: Smoking and Preoperative Advice

### Clinical Scenario

A 55-year-old man who smokes one pack of cigarettes per day is scheduled for an **inguinal hernia repair** in six weeks. He asks for advice regarding smoking and whether he should quit before the surgery.

### Question

What is the recommended preoperative advice regarding **smoking cessation** according to the **European Hernia Society (EHS)** and **American Hernia Society (AHS)** guidelines?

A) Stop smoking for 4-6 weeks
B) Stop smoking for 72 hours before surgery
C) Can continue smoking
D) Make sure he doesn't give up before surgery but make efforts to stop afterwards
E) General stop smoking advice

### Explanation

Smoking has been shown to increase the risk of **wound complications**, including **infection** and **poor healing** after surgery. The **European Hernia Society (EHS)** and **American Hernia Society (AHS)** recommend that patients who smoke should stop **4-6 weeks before surgery** to reduce the risk of postoperative complications. Smoking cessation for this duration allows for improvements in **wound healing** and **respiratory function**, reducing the likelihood of adverse outcomes.

- **Option A** is correct: The **EHS** and **AHS** recommend stopping smoking for **4-6 weeks** before surgery.

- **Option B** (72 hours) is insufficient to significantly reduce the risks associated with smoking.

- **Option C** (can continue smoking) is incorrect, as smoking increases the risk of complications.

- **Option D** (stop after surgery) is incorrect, as stopping smoking before surgery is more beneficial.

- **Option E** (general advice) is vague and does not align with the specific recommendation of stopping 4-6 weeks before surgery.

## Advanced Surgical Talk

Smoking is a well-known risk factor for **postoperative complications**, including **wound infections**, **dehiscence**, and **poor wound healing**. Smokers are also at increased risk for **respiratory complications** during and after surgery. The **EHS** and **AHS** guidelines emphasize the importance of **smoking cessation** for **4-6 weeks** before surgery to significantly reduce these risks.

During this time, patients experience improvements in **circulation**, **oxygenation**, and **immune function**, which enhance their body's ability to heal postoperatively. Even a short period of smoking cessation can improve **respiratory function** and reduce **anaesthetic risks**, making it a critical preoperative measure [1][2].

**Correct Answer: A) Stop smoking for 4-6 weeks**

## References


1. Muysoms FE, Miserez M, Berrevoet F, et al. Classification of primary and incisional abdominal wall hernias. Hernia. 2009;13(4):407-414.

2. Møller AM, Villebro N, Pedersen T, Tønnesen H. Effect of preoperative smoking intervention on postoperative complications: a randomised clinical trial. Lancet. 2002;359(9301):114-117

**Clinical Scenario**

A 45-year-old woman presents with a **3 cm umbilical hernia** and is scheduled for surgical repair. The surgeon explains that the procedure will require the use of **mesh**. The team discusses the need for **antibiotic prophylaxis** to prevent postoperative infections.

**Question**

What is the appropriate **antibiotic prophylaxis** for this patient undergoing **umbilical hernia repair** with mesh?

A) None
B) Single dose at induction
C) 3 doses post-op
D) A week of Augmentin
E) Single shot of Gentamicin

**Explanation**

In cases where **mesh** is used for **umbilical hernia repair**, the risk of infection is higher due to the introduction of a foreign material. Therefore, **antibiotic prophylaxis** is recommended to reduce the risk of **surgical site infections**. The standard recommendation is a **single dose of antibiotics** at the time of **induction** of anaesthesia, usually consisting of a **cephalosporin** or another broad-spectrum antibiotic, depending on the patient's allergies and local guidelines.

- **Option B** is correct: A **single dose at induction** is the appropriate antibiotic prophylaxis for mesh-based hernia repairs.

- **Option A** (None) is incorrect because mesh use increases infection risk.

- **Option C** (3 doses post-op) is not routinely recommended unless there are specific infection risks.

- **Option D** (A week of Augmentin) is excessive for routine prophylaxis.

- **Option E** (Single shot of Gentamicin) is not typically used as a single agent for this type of surgery.

**Advanced Surgical Talk**

For **umbilical hernia repairs** involving **mesh, antibiotic prophylaxis** is essential to minimize the risk of **surgical site infections** (SSIs), especially since mesh implantation increases susceptibility to infections. The **European Hernia Society** and **American Hernia Society** recommend a **single dose of intravenous antibiotics** given at the time of **induction of anaesthesia**. This approach has been shown to effectively reduce infection rates without the need for prolonged antibiotic courses.

The most commonly used antibiotics include **cephalosporins**, such as **cefazolin**, but the choice may vary based on local guidelines, patient allergies, and the microbial environment of the surgical centre. Postoperative antibiotics are typically unnecessary unless there are complications or signs of infection [1][2].

**Correct Answer: B) Single dose at induction**

### References

1.  Muysoms FE, Miserez M, Berrevoet F, et al. Classification of primary and incisional abdominal wall hernias. Hernia. 2009;13(4):407-414.

2.  Sanchez VM, Abi-Haidar YE, Itani KM. Mesh infection in ventral incisional hernia repair: incidence, contributing factors, and treatment. Surg Infect (Larchmt). 2011;12(3):205-210.

---

## Case 111: Small Umbilical Hernia Repair

### Clinical Scenario

A 38-year-old man presents with a **1 cm umbilical hernia** and is scheduled for surgical repair. The surgeon explains that, due to the small size of the hernia, the procedure will likely involve a **suture repair** without the need for mesh. The team discusses the need for **antibiotic prophylaxis**.

### Question

What is the appropriate **antibiotic prophylaxis** for this patient undergoing **umbilical hernia repair** without mesh?

A) None
B) Single dose at induction
C) 3 doses post-op

D) A week of Augmentin
E) Single shot of Gentamicin

**Explanation**

In cases of **small umbilical hernias** (around 1 cm in diameter) that are repaired using **suture repair** without mesh, **antibiotic prophylaxis** is generally **not required**. The risk of infection in suture-only repairs is low, and there is no foreign material, such as mesh, that could increase the infection risk. Therefore, routine use of antibiotics is not necessary in these cases unless the patient has specific risk factors or other indications for prophylaxis.

- **Option A** is correct: **No antibiotic prophylaxis** is required for small hernias repaired with sutures only.

- **Option B** (Single dose at induction) would be used if mesh were involved or if the patient had a higher risk of infection, but it is unnecessary here.

- **Option C** (3 doses post-op) is excessive for a small, simple hernia repair.

- **Option D** (A week of Augmentin) is not indicated for routine hernia repairs.

- **Option E** (Single shot of Gentamicin) is unnecessary for suture-only repairs.

**Advanced Surgical Talk**

When dealing with **small umbilical hernias** that do not require mesh, the risk of **surgical site infection (SSI)** is very low. This is why the **European Hernia Society** and most surgical guidelines recommend that **antibiotic prophylaxis** is not necessary for **suture-only repairs**. Antibiotics should be reserved for cases where there is a higher risk of infection, such as when mesh is used or in patients with comorbidities that increase their infection risk (e.g., **diabetes, immunosuppression**).

In this patient, a **suture repair** for a 1 cm hernia is a straightforward procedure with minimal risk, and additional antibiotic administration is not warranted [1][2].

Correct Answer: A) None

**References**

1. Miserez M, Peeters E, Aufenacker T, et al. The European Hernia Society guidelines on the treatment of umbilical hernia in adult patients. Hernia. 2014;18(4):387-393.

2. Sanchez VM, Abi-Haidar YE, Itani KM. Mesh infection in ventral incisional hernia repair: incidence, contributing factors, and treatment. Surg Infect (Larchmt). 2011;12(3):205-210.

## Case 112: Surgical Management of Umbilical Hernia

### Clinical Scenario

A 45-year-old woman presents with a **2 cm umbilical hernia**. After a detailed evaluation, the surgical team discusses the best approach for repair, considering the use of mesh to minimize the risk of recurrence.

### Question

What is the **optimal surgical management** for this patient with a 2 cm umbilical hernia?

A) 4 cm diameter flat mesh placed using an onlay technique
B) 4 cm diameter flat mesh placed using a sublay pre-peritoneal technique
C) 8 cm diameter flat mesh placed using an inlay technique
D) 8 cm diameter flat mesh placed using a sublay pre-peritoneal technique
E) 4 cm diameter flat mesh placed using an inlay technique

### Explanation

For **umbilical hernia repairs**, especially when the defect is between **1-4 cm**, the use of **mesh** is recommended to reduce the risk of recurrence. The mesh should be placed with a **3 cm overlap** beyond the edges of the hernia defect to ensure adequate coverage and support. The most appropriate technique in this case is to use an **8 cm diameter mesh** (2 cm defect + 3 cm overlap on each side) placed using a **sublay pre-peritoneal technique**. The **sublay technique** involves placing the mesh in the pre-peritoneal space, which is associated with lower recurrence rates compared to onlay or inlay techniques.

- **Option D** is correct: An **8 cm diameter flat mesh** placed using a **sublay pre-peritoneal technique** is the recommended approach for optimal coverage and long-term success.

- **Option A** (4 cm onlay mesh) and **Option B** (4 cm sublay mesh) provide insufficient overlap.

- **Option C** (8 cm inlay mesh) and **Option E** (4 cm inlay mesh) are less optimal because inlay meshes are placed directly in the defect without overlapping the surrounding tissue, which is associated with higher recurrence rates.

**Advanced Surgical Talk**

When managing an **umbilical hernia** with a defect size between **1-4 cm**, the **European Hernia Society guidelines** recommend using **mesh** to reduce the risk of recurrence, as primary suture repair alone may not be sufficient. The mesh should have at least a **3 cm overlap** beyond the defect size. For a **2 cm hernia**, an **8 cm diameter mesh** is ideal, with **pre-peritoneal (sublay) placement** being the preferred technique. This placement minimizes tension on the repair and decreases the risk of infection and recurrence.

The **sublay technique** involves placing the mesh between the rectus muscles and the peritoneum, providing a strong, tension-free repair. The **onlay** and **inlay** techniques, on the other hand, are associated with higher rates of recurrence and complications, making them less favorable in this context [1][2].

**Correct Answer: D) 8 cm diameter flat mesh placed using a sublay pre-peritoneal technique**

**References**


1. Miserez M, Peeters E, Aufenacker T, et al. The European Hernia Society guidelines on the treatment of umbilical hernia in adult patients. Hernia. 2014;18(4):387-393.

2. Muysoms FE, Miserez M, Berrevoet F, et al. Classification of primary and incisional abdominal wall hernias. Hernia. 2009;13(4):407-414.


---

## Case 113: Laparoscopic Repair for Umbilical Hernia

**Clinical Scenario**

A 50-year-old man with a **4 cm umbilical hernia** is scheduled for **laparoscopic repair**. The surgical team discusses the technique, including the **mesh placement** and overlap, in line with current guidelines for reducing recurrence and complications.

## Question

What is the **recommended mesh overlap** and surgical approach for a laparoscopic repair of an umbilical hernia, according to current guidelines?

A) Laparoscopic repair with 2 cm overlap
B) Laparoscopic repair with 3 cm overlap
C) Laparoscopic repair with 5 cm overlap
D) Open repair with 3 cm overlap
E) Open repair with no mesh

## Explanation

For **laparoscopic umbilical hernia repair**, guidelines recommend a **5 cm mesh overlap** beyond the edges of the defect to minimize the risk of hernia recurrence. Additionally, guidelines suggest that the **primary defect should be closed**, which helps to reduce postoperative bulging and **seroma formation**. While laparoscopic suturing can be technically challenging, it is recommended to close the defect before applying the mesh to improve outcomes. The use of **intraperitoneal onlay mesh (IPOM)** is the most commonly used technique, though **extraperitoneal approaches** are also considered viable.

- **Option C is correct:** A **laparoscopic repair with 5 cm overlap** is recommended according to guidelines.

- **Option A** (2 cm overlap) and **Option B** (3 cm overlap) provide insufficient coverage, increasing the risk of recurrence.

- **Option D** (open repair with 3 cm overlap) is not the recommended approach for a laparoscopic procedure.

- **Option E** (open repair without mesh) is inappropriate for a defect of this size, as mesh is recommended for hernia repairs larger than 1 cm.

## Advanced Surgical Talk

For **laparoscopic hernia repairs**, particularly in **ventral** or **umbilical hernias**, the use of **mesh with a 5 cm overlap** is crucial to ensure that the hernia defect is adequately covered and to reduce the risk of recurrence. A **primary closure** of the hernia defect is also advised to decrease the likelihood of postoperative complications such as **bulging** and **seroma formation**. While **intraperitoneal onlay mesh (IPOM)** is the standard approach, the **extraperitoneal technique** can also be used depending on surgeon experience and patient factors.

Laparoscopic repair offers the benefits of faster recovery and fewer wound complications compared to open repair, but it requires skill in laparoscopic suturing. Closing the defect and achieving sufficient overlap with the mesh are critical steps for a successful long-term repair [1][2].

**Correct Answer: C) Laparoscopic repair with 5 cm overlap**

## References


1.  Muysoms FE, Miserez M, Berrevoet F, et al. Classification of primary and incisional abdominal wall hernias. Hernia. 2009;13(4):407-414.

2.  Miserez M, Peeters E, Aufenacker T, et al. The European Hernia Society guidelines on the treatment of umbilical hernia in adult patients. Hernia. 2014;18(4):387-393.


---

## Case 114: Necrotizing Fasciitis

### Clinical Scenario

A 60-year-old man presents with rapidly progressing soft tissue infection, and the surgical team suspects **necrotizing fasciitis**. The patient's history reveals several potential risk factors for this severe infection.

### Question

Which of the following is the **most common predisposing risk factor** for **necrotizing fasciitis**?

A) Diabetes
B) Malnutrition
C) Azathioprine
D) Prednisolone
E) Intravenous drug use (IVDU)

### Explanation

The most common predisposing risk factor for **necrotizing fasciitis** is **diabetes mellitus**. Diabetes increases susceptibility to infections due to impaired immune function, poor circulation, and delayed wound healing. These factors create a favorable environment for the development of severe soft tissue infections such as necrotizing fasciitis.

- **Option A** is correct: **Diabetes** is the most common predisposing factor for necrotizing fasciitis.

- **Option B** (Malnutrition), **Option C** (Azathioprine), and **Option D** (Prednisolone) are potential risk factors, but diabetes is more common.

- **Option E** (Intravenous drug use) can predispose individuals to infections, but diabetes remains the leading risk factor for necrotizing fasciitis.

**Advanced Surgical Talk**

**Necrotizing fasciitis** is a life-threatening infection that rapidly destroys soft tissue and requires immediate surgical intervention. While several risk factors can predispose patients to this condition, including **immunosuppressive therapy** (such as **azathioprine** or **prednisolone**), **malnutrition**, and **intravenous drug use (IVDU)**, **diabetes** is the most common predisposing factor.

Diabetes impairs **immune response** and causes **microvascular changes** that limit tissue perfusion and oxygenation, making patients more vulnerable to severe infections. Early recognition of necrotizing fasciitis and prompt surgical debridement, along with broad-spectrum antibiotics, is crucial for improving patient outcomes [1][2].

**Correct Answer: A) Diabetes**

**References**


1.  Stevens DL, Bryant AE. Necrotizing soft-tissue infections. N Engl J Med. 2017;377(23):2253-2265.

2.  Endorf FW, Cancio LC, Klein MB. Necrotizing soft-tissue infections: clinical guidelines. J Burn Care Res. 2009;30(5):769-775.


## Case 115: Intraoperative Discovery of Colon Tumour

**Clinical Scenario**

A 50-year-old woman presents with **right iliac fossa pain** and undergoes a **laparoscopic appendicectomy**. During the procedure, a **large ascending colon tumour** is discovered involving the **right proximal ureter** and **kidney**. There are no visible metastases on the peritoneum or liver. The surgical team debates the next steps.

## Question

Given the intraoperative discovery of a large tumour involving the right proximal ureter and kidney, what is the **most appropriate next step** in the management of this patient?

A) Perform a right hemicolectomy and nephrectomy
B) Biopsy the tumour and continue with the appendicectomy
C) Call for a urology opinion and proceed with tumour resection
D) Close the patient and schedule an urgent MDT discussion
E) Perform a palliative resection of the tumour

## Explanation

In cases where an unexpected large tumour is found intraoperatively, particularly one involving vital structures such as the **ureter** and **kidney**, it is essential to halt the procedure and thoroughly assess the patient's situation before proceeding. The best approach in this scenario is to **close the patient** and discuss the findings at a **multidisciplinary team (MDT) meeting**. This allows for a comprehensive evaluation of the patient's kidney function (particularly the **contralateral kidney**), urological input, and appropriate planning of a combined surgery if necessary.

Proceeding with immediate resection without knowing the status of the **left kidney** could result in significant postoperative morbidity, including the risk of **lifelong dialysis** if the left kidney is non-functioning. The **MDT** approach also ensures that the patient is fully informed and can give consent to the most appropriate treatment plan.

- **Option D** is correct: **Closing the patient and discussing at MDT** is the most appropriate course of action.

- **Option A** (performing immediate hemicolectomy and nephrectomy) is risky without knowing the function of the other kidney.

- **Option B** (biopsy and continue) is inappropriate, as the discovery of a large tumor warrants more comprehensive evaluation.

- **Option C** (proceeding with resection) may cause unnecessary harm without full understanding of the patient's renal function and overall treatment plan.

- **Option E** (palliative resection) is not indicated, as there is no evidence of metastasis, and definitive management should be planned after discussion.

## Advanced Surgical Talk

Intraoperative discovery of a **colonic tumour** involving adjacent structures such as the **ureter** and **kidney** is a challenging situation. The **first priority** is to ensure that no irreversible decisions are made before the patient's full clinical status is evaluated, particularly their **renal function**. A key step is to assess the function of the **contralateral kidney** to avoid rendering the patient dialysis-dependent in the event of a nephrectomy.

The appropriate next step in such cases is to close the abdomen and arrange an urgent **multidisciplinary team (MDT)** meeting. This ensures input from **urology**, **oncology**, **surgical colleagues**, and **radiology**, allowing for a coordinated approach to treatment that prioritizes patient safety and consent. **Immediate surgery** may not be necessary, and in most cases, proper preoperative planning leads to better outcomes [1][2].

**Correct Answer: D) Close the patient and schedule an urgent MDT discussion**

## References


1. Biondi A, Grosso G, Mistretta A, et al. Laparoscopic vs. open approach for colorectal cancer: evolution over time of minimal invasive surgery. BMC Surg. 2013;13(Suppl 2).

2. Benson AB, Venook AP, Al-Hawary MM, et al. NCCN guidelines insights: colon cancer, version 2.2018. J Natl Compr Canc Netw. 2018;16(4):359-369


# Case 116: Classification of Obesity

## Clinical Scenario

A 45-year-old man presents to the clinic with a **BMI of 47**. The surgical team discusses his classification according to both **WHO guidelines** and **surgical literature** terminology, as this will influence the approach to his upcoming abdominal surgery.

## Question

According to the **WHO classifications** and **surgical literature**, how would you categorize a patient with a **BMI of 47**?

A) Overweight
B) Class I
C) Class II
D) Class III
E) Super obese

**Explanation**

The **World Health Organization (WHO)** classifies **obesity** based on **BMI** as follows:

- **Class I** (Obesity): BMI 30-34.9

- **Class II** (Severe obesity): BMI 35-39.9

- **Class III** (Morbid obesity): BMI ≥ 40

In **surgical literature**, a patient with a **BMI > 45** is often referred to as **super obese**. Though these patients technically fall under **Class III obesity** according to WHO classifications, surgical practice differentiates them further due to the higher risks associated with this degree of obesity.

- **Option E** is correct: A BMI of 47 qualifies the patient as **super obese** in surgical terminology.

- **Option A** (Overweight) refers to a BMI between 25-29.9, which does not apply here.

- **Option B** (Class I) refers to a BMI between 30-34.9.

- **Option C** (Class II) refers to a BMI between 35-39.9.

- **Option D** (Class III) is correct according to WHO but not detailed enough for surgical literature, which further defines **super obesity**.

**Advanced Surgical Talk**

**Obesity** is a well-known risk factor for postoperative complications, particularly in **abdominal surgery**. In **surgical literature**, special consideration is given to patients who are classified as **super obese** (BMI > 45), as they pose unique challenges in terms of anaesthesia, wound healing, and the risk of **deep vein thrombosis (DVT)** and **pulmonary complications**.

While the **WHO** categorizes all patients with a **BMI ≥ 40** as **Class III obese** (morbid obesity), surgeons typically differentiate **super obese** patients due to their substantially higher risks. This classification aids in **preoperative planning**, ensuring that the surgical team accounts for these additional factors when managing patients with extreme obesity [1][2].

**Correct Answer: E) Super obese**

## References


1.  Sturm R, Hattori A. Morbid obesity rates continue to rise rapidly in the United States. Int J Obes (Lond). 2013;37(6):889-891.

2.  Kuk JL, Ardern CI. Influence of age on the association between various measures of obesity and all-cause mortality. J Am Geriatr Soc. 2009;57(11):2077-2084


## Case 117: Guidelines for Observational Studies

### Clinical Scenario

A researcher is conducting a large-scale **observational cohort study** and wants to ensure the study follows the appropriate guidelines to improve transparency and robustness in the reporting of findings. The researcher asks which set of guidelines should be used for this type of study.

### Question

Which of the following guidelines is the correct one to follow for an **observational study**, including cohort, case-control, and cross-sectional designs?

A) CONSORT guidelines
B) PRISMA guidelines
C) STROBE guidelines
D) SQUIRE guidelines
E) CHERRIES guidelines

### Explanation

The **STROBE guidelines** (Strengthening the Reporting of Observational Studies in Epidemiology) are specifically designed to guide the reporting of **observational studies**, including **cohort**, **case-control**, and **cross-sectional studies**. These guidelines help ensure that such studies are reported with clarity and transparency, improving the reproducibility and robustness of the findings.

- **Option C is correct:** The **STROBE guidelines** apply to **observational studies**.

- **Option A** (CONSORT guidelines) applies to **randomized controlled trials (RCTs)**.

- **Option B** (PRISMA guidelines) applies to **systematic reviews and meta-analyses**.

- **Option D** (SQUIRE guidelines) applies to **quality improvement studies**.

- **Option E** (CHERRIES guidelines) applies to **web surveys**.

## Advanced Surgical Talk

When conducting and reporting on **observational studies**, the **STROBE guidelines** provide a comprehensive checklist to ensure that all critical components of the study, including **design**, **data collection**, **analysis**, and **interpretation**, are clearly presented. Following these guidelines helps researchers improve the transparency and quality of their work, making it easier for readers and reviewers to evaluate the study's validity.

The **EQUATOR network** provides an excellent resource for identifying appropriate guidelines based on the type of study being conducted, ensuring that research meets high standards of **methodological rigor**. Different guidelines cater to different types of research, such as **PRISMA** for meta-analyses and **CONSORT** for RCTs, but for **observational studies**, **STROBE** remains the gold standard [1][2].

Correct Answer: C) STROBE guidelines

## References


1. Vandenbroucke JP, von Elm E, Altman DG, et al. Strengthening the reporting of observational studies in epidemiology (STROBE): explanation and elaboration. PLoS Med. 2007;4(10).

2. Moher D, Liberati A, Tetzlaff J, Altman DG; PRISMA Group. Preferred reporting items for systematic reviews and meta-analyses: the PRISMA statement. PLoS Med. 2009;6(7).

# Case 118: Jehovah's Witness Child Requiring Blood Transfusion

## Clinical Scenario

A **15-year-old girl** presents to the emergency department after a severe trauma with significant blood loss. She is a **Jehovah's Witness**, and her parents refuse a **blood transfusion** on religious grounds. However, the patient is conscious and expresses her willingness to receive the transfusion.

## Question

What is the most appropriate next step in managing this patient, according to **Gillick/Fraser competence**?

A) Transfuse anyway
B) Don't transfuse
C) Give Albumin 20%
D) Resuscitate with crystalloid only
E) Contact the on-call solicitor and make the child ward of court

## Explanation

In this scenario, the 15-year-old patient is assessed to be **Gillick/Fraser competent**, meaning she is capable of understanding the nature and consequences of her medical treatment. According to the principle of **Gillick competence**, a minor can consent to treatment if they demonstrate sufficient maturity and understanding, even if their parents object. Since the patient has **consented** to the transfusion, it is ethically and legally appropriate to proceed with the **blood transfusion**, regardless of her parents' refusal.

- **Option A** is correct: **Transfuse anyway** in this case, as the patient has demonstrated competence and has consented to the treatment.

- **Option B** (Don't transfuse) is incorrect because the patient has consented, and not transfusing could put her life at risk.

- **Option C** (Give Albumin 20%) is not appropriate, as **albumin** is similarly objected to by many Jehovah's Witnesses, and blood transfusion is the required treatment here.

- **Option D** (Resuscitate with crystalloid only) would not be sufficient to address her severe blood loss.

- **Option E** (Make the child ward of court) is unnecessary if the patient has **consented** and is competent.

## Advanced Surgical Talk

The concept of **Gillick competence** allows a **minor** to accept medical treatment if they have sufficient understanding and intelligence to appreciate the implications of their decision. This principle applies even if the parents object to the treatment, as is the case with **Jehovah's Witnesses** and their refusal of blood transfusions on religious grounds. Importantly, while **Gillick competence** allows minors to **accept** treatment, it does not extend to their ability to **refuse life-saving treatment** in situations where they may not fully comprehend the consequences.

In cases of **Jehovah's Witnesses**, medical teams may face challenges in balancing respect for religious beliefs with the ethical obligation to provide life-saving care. If a competent minor consents to treatment, their wishes take precedence over parental objections. If the minor refuses, legal intervention may be necessary to protect the child's best interests [1][2].

Correct Answer: A) Transfuse anyway

## References


1.  Gillick v West Norfolk and Wisbech Area Health Authority [1986] AC 112.

2.  British Medical Association. Consent, rights, and choices in health care for children and young people. London: BMJ Books; 2001


---

## Case 119: TAPP Approach

### Clinical Scenario

A 58-year-old man is undergoing surgery for a **direct inguinal hernia**, and the surgeon is using a **transabdominal preperitoneal (TAPP) approach** for the repair. During the procedure, the surgeon visualizes the **inferior epigastric vessels** and the **medial umbilical ligament** to help orient themselves. There is also a potential **indirect component** to the hernia.

### Question

What is the most appropriate surgical approach for the repair of this inguinal hernia?

A) Open hernia repair
B) Transabdominal preperitoneal (TAPP) repair
C) Totally extraperitoneal (TEP) repair
D) Suture repair
E) Plug repair

## Explanation

The **transabdominal preperitoneal (TAPP) repair** is a commonly used laparoscopic technique for repairing both **direct** and **indirect inguinal hernias**. In this approach, the surgeon enters the peritoneal cavity, allowing for visualization of key anatomical landmarks such as the **inferior epigastric vessels** and **medial umbilical ligament**. This orientation is crucial for distinguishing between **direct** and **indirect** hernias and ensuring proper placement of the mesh.

- **Option B** is correct: The **TAPP approach** is appropriate for repairing a **direct inguinal hernia**, especially when there may be an indirect component.

- **Option A** (Open hernia repair) may be used but is not the first choice in this laparoscopic scenario.

- **Option C** (TEP repair) is another laparoscopic approach, but in this case, the **TAPP approach** has been chosen, which involves entering the peritoneum.

- **Option D** (Suture repair) would be inadequate for this type of hernia.

- **Option E** (Plug repair) is also inadequate for this scenario, as mesh repair is typically recommended.

## Advanced Surgical Talk

The **transabdominal preperitoneal (TAPP) approach** allows surgeons to visualize the hernia from within the abdominal cavity, making it ideal for addressing both **direct** and **indirect inguinal hernias**. By identifying the **inferior epigastric vessels** and **medial umbilical ligament**, the surgeon can correctly orient themselves and ensure accurate placement of the mesh.

The **TAPP technique** is distinguished from the **totally extraperitoneal (TEP) repair**, where the surgery is performed outside the peritoneal cavity. Both are effective, but **TAPP** provides better visualization of the anatomy, making it the preferred choice in cases with complex anatomy or uncertainty about the hernia type. The use of **mesh** ensures a tension-free repair and reduces the risk of recurrence, which is important in the long-term management of inguinal hernias [1][2].

**Correct Answer: B) Transabdominal preperitoneal (TAPP) repair**

### References


1. Miserez M, Peeters E, Aufenacker T, et al. The European Hernia Society guidelines on the treatment of inguinal hernia in adult patients. Hernia. 2014;18(4):387-393.

2. Bittner R, Schwarz J. Totally extraperitoneal inguinal hernia repair (TEP). Surg Clin North Am. 2008;88(1):115-132.


---

## Case 120: Management of Basal Cell Carcinoma

### Clinical Scenario

A 55-year-old woman presents with a **pearly white nodule** on her **trunk**, measuring less than **20mm** in diameter. The lesion is clinically consistent with a **basal cell carcinoma (BCC)**. The patient asks about the appropriate treatment and management options.

### Question

What is the most appropriate management for this **low-risk** basal cell carcinoma (BCC) on the trunk?

A) Mohs microscopic surgery
B) Wide local excision with 10mm margins
C) Topical imiquimod
D) Radiotherapy
E) Standard excision with 4mm margins

### Explanation

This lesion is a **low-risk basal cell carcinoma (BCC)** due to its size (<20mm) and location on the trunk, where BCCs are typically lower risk. The recommended treatment for low-risk BCCs on the trunk is **standard excision** with **4mm margins**. This approach ensures complete removal of the lesion while minimizing the amount of healthy tissue excised.

- **Option E** is correct: A **standard excision with 4mm margins** is appropriate for this low-risk BCC.

- **Option A** (Mohs microscopic surgery) is generally reserved for **high-risk BCCs** or lesions in cosmetically sensitive areas like the face.

- **Option B** (wide excision with 10mm margins) is excessive for a low-risk BCC.

- **Option C** (topical imiquimod) may be used for superficial BCCs but is not the first-line treatment for nodular BCCs.

- **Option D** (radiotherapy) is typically reserved for patients who are not good surgical candidates or for large, high-risk lesions.

## Advanced Surgical Talk

**Basal cell carcinoma (BCC)** is the most common type of skin cancer and is often found on **sun-exposed areas**, though lesions on the trunk are also common. The management of BCC depends on the **risk factors** of the lesion, including **size**, **location**, and **margins**. For low-risk BCCs like the one described here (on the trunk and less than 20mm), a **standard surgical excision** with **4mm margins** is the gold standard ( Table 8).

Other options, such as **Mohs surgery**, are typically reserved for high-risk cases, particularly in **cosmetically sensitive areas** like the face, where tissue conservation is critical. **Topical treatments** like **imiquimod** are used for **superficial BCCs**, but for nodular lesions, surgical excision is the preferred approach. **Radiotherapy** is often used for older patients or those who are not fit for surgery, but it is not typically first-line treatment for low-risk cases [1][2].

**Correct Answer: E) Standard excision with 4mm margins**

## References


1. Telfer NR, Colver GB, Morton CA; British Association of Dermatologists. Guidelines for the management of basal cell carcinoma. Br J Dermatol. 2008;159(1):35-48.

2. Kauvar ANB, Cronin T Jr, Roenigk R, et al. Consensus for nonmelanoma skin cancer treatment: basal cell carcinoma, including a cost analysis of treatment methods. Dermatol Surg. 2015;41(5):550-571.

*Table 8: Patient Management Pathway - Basal Cell Carcinoma*

| Scenario | Pathway Description | Treatment Options |
| --- | --- | --- |
| Low-risk BCC, GP competent and facility suitable | GP can treat surgically or refer to MDT (if necessary) | Surgical excision |
| High-risk BCC, or low-risk BCC and GP not competent | Refer to Skin Cancer MDT | Standard surgical excision or Mohs surgery, depending on MDT decision |
| Low-risk BCC, presenting to Skin Cancer MDT | MDT discusses management options and decides on appropriate treatment | Standard excision, topical therapies (e.g., imiquimod), cryotherapy, photodynamic therapy, or radiotherapy |
| High-risk BCC, suitable for surgical excision | MDT recommends standard excision or Mohs surgery | Surgical excision with adequate margins or Mohs micrographic surgery |
| High-risk BCC, patient not suitable for surgery | MDT discusses non-surgical options (due to age, comorbidities, or other factors) | Vismodegib for advanced cases, or other treatments depending on patient's condition |

## Case 121: Basal Cell Carcinoma in a High-Risk Area

### Clinical Scenario

A 62-year-old man presents with a **basal cell carcinoma (BCC)** on his **neck** that is **less than 20mm** in diameter. The lesion is located in a **high-risk area** and the surgical team discusses the most appropriate management, considering the need for wider margins due to the location.

## Question

What is the most appropriate management for this **high-risk** basal cell carcinoma (BCC) on the neck?

A) Excise with 4mm margins
B) Mohs micrographic surgery
C) Excise with 5mm margins
D) Radiotherapy
E) Topical imiquimod

## Explanation

In the management of **basal cell carcinoma (BCC)**, the **location** of the lesion significantly impacts the recommended treatment approach. **High-risk areas** include the **neck**, face, and other cosmetically or functionally sensitive regions. For BCCs located in high-risk areas, the recommended margin is **5mm**, even if the lesion is less than 20mm in diameter.

While **Mohs micrographic surgery** may be considered, it is generally reserved for cases with **ill-defined margins** or **recurrent** lesions. In this case, **standard excision with 5mm margins** is the first-line treatment, unless there are additional risk factors.

- **Option C** is correct: Excising with **5mm margins** is recommended due to the high-risk location.

- **Option A** (4mm margins) is used for low-risk BCCs in non-critical areas.

- **Option B** (Mohs micrographic surgery) may be considered if the lesion has **ill-defined margins**, but standard excision is preferred here.

- **Option D** (Radiotherapy) is generally reserved for cases where surgery is not an option.

- **Option E** (Topical imiquimod) is used for superficial BCCs and not typically recommended for nodular BCCs in high-risk areas.

## Advanced Surgical Talk

**Basal cell carcinomas (BCCs)** located in **high-risk areas**, such as the neck, require wider excision margins compared to BCCs in low-risk areas. This is because the risk of recurrence is higher, and achieving **clear margins** is essential to reduce the chance of the lesion returning. For lesions in high-risk areas, **5mm margins** are recommended, even for small tumours (<20mm).

In cases where there are additional risk factors, such as **ill-defined borders**, or in cases of recurrent BCC, **Mohs micrographic surgery** may be considered. This technique allows for the precise removal of the tumour while sparing as much healthy tissue as possible. However, for most primary BCCs in high-risk areas, **standard surgical excision** with 5mm margins remains the first-line approach [1][2].

**Correct Answer: C) Excise with 5mm margins**

### References

1.  Telfer NR, Colver GB, Morton CA; British Association of Dermatologists. Guidelines for the management of basal cell carcinoma. Br J Dermatol. 2008;159(1):35-48.

2.  Kauvar ANB, Cronin T Jr, Roenigk R, et al. Consensus for nonmelanoma skin cancer treatment: basal cell carcinoma, including a cost analysis of treatment methods. Dermatol Surg. 2015;41(5):550-571.

## Case 122: Management of Squamous Cell Carcinoma

### Clinical Scenario

A 45-year-old woman with **stable HIV** presents with a lesion on her **forearm**. On examination, the lesion has **raised hard edges** and a **necrotic centre**, consistent with a **squamous cell carcinoma (SCC)**. The lesion is small and considered a **T1 tumour**.

### Question

What is the most appropriate **surgical margin** for excision of this squamous cell carcinoma (SCC) in a patient with **HIV**?

A) Standard excision with 4mm margins
B) Standard excision with 2mm margins
C) Mohs micrographic surgery
D) Excision with 6mm margins
E) Radiotherapy

### Explanation

In cases of **squamous cell carcinoma (SCC)**, the standard recommendation for **T1 tumours** (tumours smaller than 2cm with low-risk features) is to excise with **4mm margins**. However, in patients who are **immunocompromised**, such as those with **HIV**, a larger margin is often recommended due to the increased risk of **recurrence** and **metastasis**. In this case, a **6mm margin** is appropriate to ensure complete excision and to reduce the risk of recurrence in the setting of immunosuppression.

- **Option D** is correct: Excision with **6mm margins** is recommended for **immunocompromised** patients, including those with HIV.

- **Option A** (4mm margins) would be used for **immunocompetent** patients with T1 tumours.

- **Option B** (2mm margins) is insufficient for SCC.

- **Option C** (Mohs micrographic surgery) may be used in high-risk cases or for lesions in cosmetically sensitive areas, but it is not the first-line treatment here.

- **Option E** (Radiotherapy) is generally reserved for patients who are not candidates for surgery or for more advanced cases.

## Advanced Surgical Talk

**Squamous cell carcinoma (SCC)** is the second most common type of skin cancer and often presents as a **scaly, ulcerated** lesion with **hard edges**. Treatment depends on the size, depth, and risk factors of the lesion. In patients who are **immunocompromised**, such as those with **HIV**, the risk of **recurrence** and **metastasis** is higher, and **wider excision margins** are required.

For **T1 SCCs** in **immunocompetent** patients, the standard treatment is excision with **4mm margins**. However, in immunocompromised patients, wider margins, such as **6mm**, are recommended to reduce the risk of incomplete excision and recurrence. **Mohs surgery** may be considered in cases where there are ill-defined margins or for high-risk areas, but it is not necessary for straightforward T1 lesions unless additional risk factors are present [1][2].

Correct Answer: D) Excision with 6mm margins

## References

1. Stratigos AJ, Garbe C, Lebbe C, et al. European interdisciplinary guideline on invasive squamous cell carcinoma of the skin: part 1. Epidemiology, diagnostics and prevention. Eur J Cancer. 2020;128:60-82.

2. Motaparthi K, Kapil JP, Velazquez EF. Histologic mimics of squamous cell carcinoma. Dermatol Clin. 2019;37(3):315-331.

## Case 123: Suspected Malignant Melanoma

### Clinical Scenario

A 48-year-old woman presents with a **small, pigmented lesion** on her **forearm** that has been changing in appearance over the past few months. The lesion shows **asymmetry**, **irregular borders**, and **different shades** of black and brown. The surgical team suspects a **malignant melanoma** and discusses the next steps for assessment and management.

### Question

What is the most appropriate **initial assessment** and management step for this suspected **malignant melanoma**?

A) Immediate wide excision
B) Observation without further intervention
C) Clinical photography and surgical excision
D) Shave biopsy
E) Cryotherapy

### Explanation

In cases where **malignant melanoma** is suspected, the **first step** involves clinical assessment, often using the **ABCD criteria** (Asymmetry, irregular Borders, Colour variation, and Diameter). For documentation and baseline comparison, **clinical photography** is important. Following this, the lesion should be **surgically excised** with narrow margins for **histopathological examination** to confirm the diagnosis and guide further management.

- **Option C is correct:** **Clinical photography** should be taken for baseline documentation, followed by **surgical excision** with narrow margins for histopathological confirmation.

- **Option A** (Immediate wide excision) is not recommended as the first step. Initial excision should be done with narrow margins.

- **Option B** (Observation without intervention) is inappropriate for suspected malignant melanoma, where early diagnosis and treatment are essential.

- **Option D** (Shave biopsy) is not suitable for melanoma, as this can compromise histological depth assessment.

- **Option E** (Cryotherapy) is not appropriate for melanoma, which requires surgical excision.

## Advanced Surgical Talk

**Malignant melanoma**, or simply **melanoma**, is one of the most aggressive forms of skin cancer. Early detection and treatment are crucial for improving patient outcomes. **Clinical photography** plays an important role in documenting the lesion for future comparison, particularly if any observation or follow-up is planned. However, for suspected melanoma, **surgical excision** with **narrow margins** (e.g., 1-2 mm) is the gold standard for obtaining a **histopathological diagnosis**.

The **ABCD criteria**—Asymmetry, Border irregularity, Colour variation, and Diameter greater than 6 mm—are useful for clinical assessment. A confirmed melanoma diagnosis will guide further treatment, including **wide excision** with appropriate margins, which depends on the **Breslow thickness** of the tumour. Early and accurate diagnosis is key to reducing morbidity and improving survival rates [1][2].

Correct Answer: C) Clinical photography and surgical excision

## References


1. Bastian BC. The molecular pathology of melanoma: an integrated taxonomy of melanocytic neoplasia. Annu Rev Pathol. 2014;9:239-271.

2. Coit DG, Thompson JA, Albertini MR, et al. Melanoma, version 2.2016, NCCN clinical practice guidelines in oncology. J Natl Compr Canc Netw. 2016;14(4):450-473.

## Clinical Scenario

A 52-year-old woman presents after excision of a **stage IA melanoma**. The lesion was less than 1mm thick, without ulceration, and no lymph node involvement was suspected. The patient inquires about the appropriate follow-up and whether further staging investigations are required.

## Question

What is the most appropriate **management** and **follow-up** for this patient with **stage IA melanoma**?

A) Sentinel lymph node biopsy
B) Adjuvant radiotherapy
C) Re-excision with 2 cm margins
D) Reassurance and surveillance only
E) Systemic chemotherapy

## Explanation

For **stage IA melanoma** (tumour thickness ≤1 mm, without ulceration or lymph node involvement), the recommended management is **reassurance** and **surveillance**. Sentinel lymph node biopsy and staging investigations are **not** required for **stage IA melanoma**. Follow-up typically involves **3-6 monthly surveillance** for the first year, and patients are advised on **self-examination**. Regular surveillance helps detect any recurrence or new primary melanomas early.

- **Option D** is correct: **Reassurance and surveillance** are appropriate for stage IA disease.

- **Option A** (Sentinel lymph node biopsy) is unnecessary in stage IA melanoma.

- **Option B** (Adjuvant radiotherapy) is used only in advanced stages of melanoma.

- **Option C** (Re-excision with 2 cm margins) is excessive; **1 cm margins** are appropriate for stage I melanoma.

- **Option E** (Systemic chemotherapy) is used in more advanced melanoma stages, not in stage IA.

**Advanced Surgical Talk**

**Stage IA melanoma** is classified based on the **American Joint Committee on Cancer (AJCC)** guidelines, which consider **tumour thickness** and the absence of **ulceration** or lymph node involvement. For **stage IA melanoma**, the risk of recurrence or metastasis is low, and **surveillance** is the mainstay of management. The typical follow-up protocol includes **3-6 monthly reviews** for the first **12 months**, with a focus on detecting any recurrence or new melanomas.

Patients should be educated on **self-examination** to monitor for any suspicious changes in their skin. Checking **vitamin D levels** preoperatively is common practice, as melanoma patients may be at risk for deficiency, particularly if advised to avoid sun exposure.

For **stage I melanomas**, excision with **1 cm margins** is recommended, and more extensive surgical margins (e.g., 2 cm) are reserved for thicker lesions classified as **stage II or III. Sentinel lymph node biopsy** and other staging investigations are generally unnecessary unless there are higher-risk features [1][2].

Correct Answer: D) Reassurance and surveillance only

**References**

1.  Bastian BC. The molecular pathology of melanoma: an integrated taxonomy of melanocytic neoplasia. Annu Rev Pathol. 2014;9:239-271.

2.  Coit DG, Thompson JA, Albertini MR, et al. Melanoma, version 2.2016, NCCN clinical practice guidelines in oncology. J Natl Compr Canc Netw. 2016;14(4):450-473.

## Case 125: Importance of Attention to Detail

### Clinical Scenario

During a high-pressure situation in the operating room, a medication is about to be administered to a patient undergoing a critical procedure. The surgical assistant hands the vial to the surgeon without checking the **expiry date** of the drug. The surgeon, in the rush of the moment, considers administering the drug without verifying its expiration status.

### Question

What is the most appropriate course of action in this scenario?

A) Administer the drug if it appears fine
B) Ask the assistant to administer the drug
C) Verify the expiry date of the drug before administration
D) Administer the drug but document it
E) Proceed and notify the team afterward

**Explanation**

The **responsibility** for ensuring patient safety during medical procedures lies with every team member, but ultimately, the **surgeon** or physician administering the drug must verify that it is safe for use. This includes checking the **expiry date** of the drug. Administering an expired drug can have serious consequences, including reduced efficacy or potential harm to the patient. The question underscores the importance of **attention to detail** and highlights that sometimes, the simplest steps, such as verifying the expiry date, can prevent serious complications.

- **Option C** is correct: Always **verify the expiry date** of the drug before administering it to ensure patient safety.

- **Option A** (Administer the drug if it appears fine) is incorrect because the appearance of a drug does not guarantee its safety.

- **Option B** (Ask the assistant to administer the drug) is inappropriate; as the physician in charge, the responsibility lies with you.

- **Option D** (Administer the drug but document it) is not an acceptable course of action because it bypasses the verification step.

- **Option E** (Proceed and notify the team afterward) is dangerous and unprofessional, as it could expose the patient to unnecessary risk.

**Advanced Surgical Talk**

In any medical or surgical procedure, **patient safety** is paramount. Ensuring that drugs are administered properly and are within their **expiration date** is a basic but crucial task that must never be overlooked. **Attention to detail** is vital, particularly in high-stakes environments where simple oversights can lead to preventable errors. By always checking the expiry date and verifying the safety of any medication, medical professionals can avoid critical mistakes.

This scenario also emphasizes the importance of remaining **vigilant** and not becoming complacent, especially in routine tasks. Every detail matters, and paying attention to even the smallest aspect of patient care can make the difference between a good outcome and a critical failure [1][2].

**Correct Answer: C) Verify the expiry date of the drug before administration**

### References

1. Reason J. Human error: models and management. BMJ. 2000;320(7237):768-770.

2. Kohn LT, Corrigan JM, Donaldson MS. To err is human: building a safer health system. Washington, DC: National Academy Press; 2000.

## Case 126: Large Inguinoscrotal Hernia

### Clinical Scenario

A 32-year-old man presents with a **very large inguinoscrotal hernia**. Upon imaging, it is revealed that part of his **stomach** is within the hernia, which is extremely rare. The surgical team discusses the potential complications, including the likelihood of **losing his testicle** as part of the procedure.

### Question

What is the most important issue to address when counselling this patient regarding the potential loss of a testicle during the procedure?

A) Postoperative infection
B) Infertility risk
C) Loss of libido
D) Cosmetic disfigurement
E) Psychological impact of testicular loss

### Explanation

The **psychological impact** of **losing a testicle** is a significant consideration, particularly in a **young man**. Although losing one testicle does not typically result in **infertility**, as the remaining testicle is usually sufficient to produce sperm, the loss can have substantial **emotional** and **psychological effects**. The patient should be thoroughly counselled about the potential for this outcome, as well as the possibility of **sperm banking** if there are concerns about fertility. If there is any **undiagnosed issue** with the remaining testicle, the patient may be at risk of **infertility** and should be offered appropriate counselling.

- **Option E** is correct: The **psychological impact** of losing a testicle, particularly in a young man, should be carefully addressed.

- **Option B** (Infertility risk) is less likely, as the remaining testicle typically compensates unless there are pre-existing issues with the other testicle.

- **Option A** (Postoperative infection) is a general concern but not specific to the loss of a testicle.

- **Option C** (Loss of libido) is incorrect, as losing one testicle does not typically affect **testosterone production** or libido.

- **Option D** (Cosmetic disfigurement) may be a concern, but the psychological impact is more significant in this case.

## Advanced Surgical Talk

In cases of **large inguinoscrotal hernias** with testicular involvement, it is crucial to counsel the patient about the potential complications, including the risk of losing the **testicle**. While **infertility** is unlikely due to the compensatory function of the remaining testicle, the **psychological** and **emotional impact** of losing a testicle can be profound, particularly in younger men. Preoperative counselling should include discussions about the potential for **sperm banking** if there are concerns about fertility.

Patients should also be informed that the loss of a single testicle typically does not affect **hormone production** or **libido**. However, addressing concerns about **self-image** and **psychological well-being** is critical to ensure the patient is fully prepared for the potential outcomes of the surgery [1][2].

Correct Answer: E) Psychological impact of testicular loss

## References


1. Ferzli GS, Edwards ED. Laparoscopic hernia repair in men: potential effects on fertility and sexuality. Hernia. 2006;10(1):20-25.

2. Lynch CD, West BT, Whitcomb BW, et al. The impact of varicocele and inguinal hernia repair on semen parameters. Urology. 2012;79(1):122-126.

## Clinical Scenario

A study is conducted to assess the **sensitivity** of a **CT scan** in detecting **colorectal lesions**, with **colonoscopy** serving as the **gold standard**. The results indicate that there were **2 true positives** (lesions detected by both CT and colonoscopy) and **3 false negatives** (lesions missed by the CT scan but detected by colonoscopy).

## Question

What is the **sensitivity** of the CT scan in detecting colorectal lesions?

A) 20%
B) 40%
C) 60%
D) 80%
E) 100%

## Explanation

**Sensitivity** measures the ability of a test to correctly identify individuals with the disease (true positives) out of all those who actually have the disease (true positives + false negatives). It is calculated using the formula:

Sensitivity=True Positives/True Positives + False Negatives

In this case:

- **True Positives (TP)** = 2 (lesions detected by both CT and colonoscopy)

- **False Negatives (FN)** = 3 (lesions missed by CT but detected by colonoscopy)

Thus, the **sensitivity** is:

Sensitivity=2/2+3=2/5=0.40 or 40%

## Advanced Surgical Talk

**Sensitivity** is an important metric for evaluating the performance of diagnostic tests, particularly in identifying diseases such as **colorectal cancer**. In this case, the **CT scan** identified **2 true positives** out of the **5 total cases** that were confirmed by colonoscopy, resulting in a sensitivity of **40%**. A low sensitivity indicates that the CT scan is missing a significant proportion of cases, which could lead to **false reassurance** and missed diagnoses.

**Colonoscopy** remains the **gold standard** for detecting colorectal lesions due to its higher sensitivity and the ability to both visualize and biopsy suspicious lesions. However, **CT scans** may still play a role in situations where colonoscopy is not feasible or in assessing disease spread beyond the colon [1][2].

Correct Answer: B) 40%

### References

1. Rex DK, et al. Quality indicators for colonoscopy. Gastrointest Endosc. 2015;81(1):31-53.

2. Pickhardt PJ, Kim DH. Colorectal cancer screening with CT colonography (virtual colonoscopy): current status and future directions. Gastroenterology. 2010;138(3):1287-1302.

---

## Case 128: Calculating Specificity for a Test

### Clinical Scenario

A diagnostic test is being evaluated for its ability to **rule out** colorectal lesions. In this case, there were **25 true negatives** (cases where both the test and the gold standard indicated no lesion) and **5 false positives** (cases where the test indicated a lesion, but the gold standard did not).

### Question

What is the **specificity** of this diagnostic test?

A) 60%
B) 70%
C) 80%
D) 83%
E) 90%

### Explanation

**Specificity** measures the ability of a test to correctly identify individuals **without** the disease (true negatives) out of all those who **do not have** the disease (true negatives + false positives). It is calculated using the formula:

Specificity=True Negatives/True Negatives +False Positives

In this case:

- **True Negatives (TN)** = 25

- **False Positives (FP)** = 5

Thus, the **specificity** is:

Specificity=25/25+5=25/30=0.833 or 83.3%

**Advanced Surgical Talk**

**Specificity** is an important diagnostic measure that tells us how well a test identifies those who **do not** have a disease. In this example, the test correctly identified 25 people who were **true negatives**, and there were 5 **false positives**. A specificity of **83%** means that the test is quite reliable at ruling out disease, though there is still some risk of **false positives**, which can lead to unnecessary further investigations or anxiety for the patient.

It is important to balance **specificity** with **sensitivity** depending on the clinical scenario. In diseases where false positives carry a higher risk (such as unnecessary surgery), a high specificity is crucial to reduce false positives. Conversely, in cases where missing a diagnosis is more dangerous (such as cancer screening), **sensitivity** may take priority [1][2].

**Correct Answer: D) 83%**

**References**


1. Bossuyt PM, Reitsma JB, Bruns DE, et al. STARD 2015: an updated list of essential items for reporting diagnostic accuracy studies. BMJ. 2015;351.

2. Parikh R, Mathai A, Parikh S, et al. Understanding and using sensitivity, specificity, and predictive values. Indian J Ophthalmol. 2008;56(1):45-50.


## Case 129: Calculating Positive Predictive Value

**Clinical Scenario**

A study is conducted to assess the performance of an **ultrasound** test in detecting **bile duct stones**. The **gold standard** for diagnosing bile duct stones is **MRCP** (Magnetic Resonance Cholangiopancreatography). Out of a sample size of **100 patients**, 50% (50 patients) have stones detected by **MRCP**. It is known that

**25 patients are true positives** (correctly identified by both ultrasound and MRCP).

## Question

What is the **positive predictive value (PPV)** of the ultrasound test in detecting bile duct stones, and how many patients would undergo an **unnecessary cholangiogram** due to **false positives**?

A) 50%
B) 75%
C) 25%
D) 60%
E) 40%

## Explanation

The **positive predictive value (PPV)** is the probability that patients who test **positive** for bile duct stones by the ultrasound **actually have the disease**, confirmed by the **gold standard** (MRCP). It is calculated using the formula:

PPV=True Positives (TP)/True Positives (TP)+False Positives (FP)

In this case:

- **True Positives (TP)** = 25 (patients who were positive for stones on both ultrasound and MRCP).

- **Total Positives** (based on ultrasound test) = 50, since 50% of the sample is expected to have stones according to MRCP.

- Since **25 patients** are true positives, the remaining **25 patients** must be **false positives** (patients who tested positive on ultrasound but were negative on MRCP).

Thus, the **PPV** is:

PPV=25/25+25=25/50=0.50 or 50%

Since **25 patients** are **false positives**, these patients may undergo **unnecessary cholangiograms**.

## Advanced Surgical Talk

In this scenario, **positive predictive value (PPV)** is essential because it indicates the likelihood that a patient who tests positive for **bile duct stones** on ultrasound **actually has stones**, confirmed by MRCP. A **PPV of 50%** means that only half of the patients who test positive will genuinely have the disease, while the other half (**false positives**) will undergo **unnecessary procedures** like cholangiograms.

The importance of **PPV** in clinical practice lies in minimizing unnecessary interventions, especially when a false positive result could lead to invasive procedures. In this case, 25 out of the 50 patients who tested positive on ultrasound were **false positives**, meaning that half of these patients would undergo unnecessary cholangiograms, which carry risks of complications [1][2].

**Correct Answer: A) 50%**

### References


1.  Parikh R, Mathai A, Parikh S, et al. Understanding and using sensitivity, specificity, and predictive values. Indian J Ophthalmol. 2008;56(1):45-50.

2.  Bossuyt PM, Reitsma JB, Bruns DE, et al. STARD 2015: an updated list of essential items for reporting diagnostic accuracy studies. BMJ. 2015;351.


## Case 130: Sensitivity and PPV

### Clinical Scenario

A study is assessing the use of **intraoperative ultrasound (USS)** to detect **common bile duct (CBD) stones**. In a sample of **100 patients**, it is known that **50 patients (50%)** have CBD stones, confirmed by **MRI**. The sensitivity and positive predictive value (PPV) of intraoperative USS for detecting stones are both **50%**.

### Question

Given that the **sensitivity** and **positive predictive value (PPV)** of intraoperative USS are **50%**, how many patients in this sample would undergo an **unnecessary cholangiogram**?

A)  50
B)  25
C)  30
D)  100
E)  None of above

### Explanation

The **sensitivity** of a test refers to its ability to correctly identify **true positives** (patients with stones), while the **positive predictive**

**value (PPV)** tells us the likelihood that a positive test result is truly indicative of the disease.

## Step 1: Calculate the True Positives and False Negatives

- **Sensitivity** is 50%, so the test correctly identifies **50%** of the patients with stones.

- Out of the 50 patients who truly have CBD stones (confirmed by MRI), the test will identify:

True Positives (TP)=50%×50=25 patients.

The remaining **25 patients** who actually have CBD stones but are **missed** by the test are **false negatives**.

## Step 2: Calculate the Total Number of Positive Test Results

- The **positive predictive value (PPV)** is 50%, meaning that 50% of the patients who test positive actually have CBD stones.

- Since **25 true positives** were identified by the test and this represents **50% of the total positive tests**, the total number of positive test results must be:

Total Positive Tests=25/50%=50 patients

## Step 3: Calculate the False Positives

- Out of the **50 total positive tests, 25 are true positives** (patients who truly have stones).

- The remaining **25 patients** who tested positive but **do not actually have CBD stones** (based on MRI) are **false positives**.

## Step 4: Determine the Number of Unnecessary Cholangiograms

- The **false positive patients** are the ones who would undergo an **unnecessary cholangiogram**. Therefore, the number of patients undergoing an unnecessary procedure due to a false positive result is **25**.

## Answer

- **25 patients** would undergo an **unnecessary cholangiogram** due to **false positive results**.

**Summary:**

Given a **sensitivity** and **PPV** of 50%, out of **100 patients** (50% of whom have confirmed CBD stones), **25 patients** would undergo unnecessary cholangiograms due to false positive results on the intraoperative ultrasound.

**Correct Answer: 25 patients**

---

## Case 131: Choosing Between Fixed or Random Effects Model in Meta-Analysis

### Clinical Scenario

You are conducting a **meta-analysis** to combine data from multiple studies that assess the outcomes of a particular treatment. The demographic data from the studies show **significant differences** between the populations, suggesting **heterogeneity**. Despite this, you are considering whether to use a **fixed** or **random effects model** for the analysis.

### Question

What is the most appropriate **statistical model** to use for this meta-analysis, given the clinical and demographic heterogeneity among the studies?

A) Fixed effects model
B) Random effects model
C) Do not perform summative analysis
D) Fixed effects model with adjustment for heterogeneity
E) Use only individual study data

### Explanation

In a **meta-analysis**, the choice between a **fixed effects** and **random effects** model depends on the degree of **heterogeneity** among the included studies. A **fixed effects model** assumes that all studies estimate the same underlying effect, which is appropriate when the studies are similar in design, population, and methodology. However, in this scenario, there is significant **heterogeneity** among the studies (e.g., differences in demographics), which suggests that the treatment effect might vary across studies.

A **random effects model** accounts for this variability by allowing each study to estimate its own effect size, which is then combined into an overall estimate. Given the **significant clinical and demographic differences** in the studies, a **random effects**

**model** is the appropriate choice, even if objective measures like $I^2$ or **Chi(Q)** do not indicate substantial heterogeneity.

- **Option B** is correct: A **random effects model** should be used due to the heterogeneity between the studies.

- **Option A** (Fixed effects model) is inappropriate in the presence of significant heterogeneity.

- **Option C** (Do not perform summative analysis) might be considered if heterogeneity is too extreme, but this scenario still allows for random effects modelling.

- **Option D** (Fixed effects model with adjustment) does not fully account for heterogeneity like a random effects model does.

- **Option E** (Use only individual study data) is not necessary, as a random effects model can provide an overall estimate despite the heterogeneity.

## Advanced Surgical Talk

When conducting a **meta-analysis**, choosing between **fixed** or **random effects models** is crucial to obtaining meaningful results. A **fixed effects model** assumes that the treatment effect is the same across all studies, which may not be appropriate when there is **significant heterogeneity**. In contrast, a **random effects model** allows for differences in treatment effects across studies, accounting for variations in study populations, methodologies, or interventions.

In cases like this, where there are substantial **clinical differences** (e.g., demographic discrepancies), a **random effects model** is the best approach, even if **objective measures of heterogeneity** (such as $I^2$ or **Chi(Q)**) do not indicate extreme variability. The **random effects model** provides a more conservative estimate of the overall effect size, incorporating both within-study and between-study variability [1][2].

**Correct Answer: B) Random effects model**

## References


1. Higgins JPT, Thompson SG, Deeks JJ, Altman DG. Measuring inconsistency in meta-analyses. BMJ. 2003;327(7414):557-560.

2.  DerSimonian R, Laird N. Meta-analysis in clinical trials. Control Clin Trials. 1986;7(3):177-188.

## Case 131: Fixed vs. Random Effects Model in Meta-Analysis

### Clinical Scenario

A meta-analysis is being conducted to assess the outcomes of various studies on a specific clinical intervention. During the analysis, significant **heterogeneity** is observed in the **demographic data** across studies, as evidenced by significant **p-values**. The research team discusses whether to use a **fixed effects model** or a **random effects model** for the analysis.

### Question

Given the observed **heterogeneity** and the significant differences in demographic data, what is the most appropriate model to use in this meta-analysis?

A) Fixed effects model
B) Random effects model
C) Summative analysis without any model
D) Perform no analysis due to heterogeneity
E) Use both fixed and random effects models simultaneously

### Explanation

The decision to use a **fixed** or **random effects** model in meta-analysis depends on the presence or absence of **heterogeneity** between the studies being analyzed:

- A **fixed effects model** assumes that all studies are estimating the same underlying effect, and differences between studies are due to chance.

- A **random effects model** assumes that there is variability between studies, and each study is estimating a different effect size. This model is appropriate when there is significant **clinical heterogeneity**, such as differences in **demographic data** or **study populations**.

In this case, the **p-values** indicate significant **heterogeneity** in the **demographic data**, suggesting that the outcomes of the studies may not be directly comparable. Therefore, a **random effects model** is the appropriate choice, as it accounts for this **variability** and provides a more conservative estimate of the overall effect size.

- **Option B** is correct: A **random effects model** should be used due to the significant heterogeneity.

- **Option A** (Fixed effects model) is inappropriate because it assumes that all studies are measuring the same effect, which is not the case here.

- **Option C** (Summative analysis without any model) is not recommended when heterogeneity exists.

- **Option D** (Perform no analysis) is overly cautious; the heterogeneity can be accounted for using the random effects model.

- **Option E** (Use both models simultaneously) is not a typical approach in meta-analysis.

## Advanced Surgical Talk

In **meta-analysis**, the choice between **fixed** and **random effects models** is critical in determining how **study differences** are accounted for. When there is **significant heterogeneity** between the studies—whether due to **clinical differences**, **study designs**, or **patient populations**—a **random effects model** is generally preferred. This model assumes that the true effect size varies between studies and provides a **weighted average** that takes this variability into account.

The $I^2$ **statistic** and **Chi-squared (Q) test** are commonly used to assess heterogeneity, but even without formal measures, the presence of **clinically significant differences** (such as demographic discrepancies) warrants the use of a **random effects model**. This approach prevents the inappropriate aggregation of disparate studies and avoids the common pitfall of **"comparing apples with oranges."** The random effects model gives a more cautious, generalized estimate that reflects the diversity across studies [1][2].

Correct Answer: B) Random effects model

## References


1. DerSimonian R, Laird N. Meta-analysis in clinical trials. Control Clin Trials. 1986;7(3):177-188.

2. Higgins JPT, Thompson SG. Quantifying heterogeneity in a meta-analysis. Stat Med. 2002;21(11):1539-1558.

## Clinical Scenario

A study is conducted comparing **MRI** and **ultrasound (USS)** for diagnosing **appendicitis** in children. A total of **20 patients** were recruited. The results show:

- **4 patients** were correctly identified as having appendicitis by **both MRI and USS**.

- **1 additional patient** was diagnosed with appendicitis on **MRI** but was **missed by USS**.

- On follow-up, **MRI** correctly identified all appendicitis cases, while **USS** missed some.

## Question

What is the **specificity** of **ultrasound (USS)** in diagnosing appendicitis in this study?

## Explanation

**Specificity** measures the ability of a test to correctly identify patients **without the disease** (true negatives) out of all patients who truly do not have the disease (true negatives + false positives). The calculation is:

Specificity=True Negatives (TN)/True Negatives (TN)+False Positives (FP)

## Step 1: Determine Total Cases

- **Total patients** = 20

- **Total cases of appendicitis (as identified by MRI)** = 5 (4 detected by both MRI and USS, and 1 detected only by MRI)

## Step 2: Determine True Negatives and False Positives for USS

- **True Negatives (TN)**: Patients who do not have appendicitis and were correctly identified by USS.

    - Total non-appendicitis cases = 20 - 5 = 15

    - Since USS did not diagnose appendicitis in the missed patient (correctly identifying them as non-appendicitis), these 15 patients are **true negatives**.

- **False Positives (FP)**: Patients without appendicitis who were incorrectly identified by USS as having appendicitis.
    - o In this scenario, USS did not report any **false positives** (all appendicitis cases diagnosed by USS were correct, and there were no over-diagnoses).

**Step 3: Calculate Specificity**

Specificity=True Negatives (TN)/True Negatives (TN)+False Positives (FP)=15/15+0=15/15=1.0 or 100%

The **specificity** of **ultrasound (USS)** in this study is **100%**, as it correctly identified all patients who did **not** have appendicitis.

**Correct Answer: 100% Specificity**

---

## Case 133: Publication Bias in Meta-Analysis

### Clinical Scenario

A meta-analysis is conducted involving **15 studies**, and the researchers are evaluating the presence of **publication bias**. A **funnel plot** is created to visually assess bias, and the **Egger test** is used to statistically assess it. The **Egger test** shows a **borderline p-value** around **0.05**, leading the research team to discuss the interpretation of publication bias.

### Question

What is the most appropriate interpretation of the **Egger test** and **funnel plot** findings in this scenario?

A) Publication bias is definitely present
B) Publication bias is definitely absent
C) The results suggest possible publication bias, but the evidence is not definitive
D) The number of studies is too small to assess publication bias
E) Funnel plots are not reliable for assessing publication bias in meta-analysis

### Explanation

**Publication bias** is typically assessed using **funnel plots** and statistical tests like the **Egger test**. When the **Egger test** shows a **p-value** of less than **0.05**, publication bias is usually considered

**significant**. However, in this scenario, the **p-value** is borderline, suggesting that the evidence for publication bias is **inconclusive**. Given that there are more than **10 studies**, it is appropriate to assess publication bias, but the **borderline p-value** means that a definitive conclusion should be avoided.

- **Option C** is correct: The results suggest **possible publication bias**, but the evidence is not definitive due to the borderline p-value.

- **Option A** (Publication bias is definitely present) is too strong a statement based on a borderline result.

- **Option B** (Publication bias is definitely absent) is also inappropriate given the borderline p-value.

- **Option D** (The number of studies is too small) is incorrect because **more than 10 studies** were included, which is sufficient for assessing publication bias.

- **Option E** (Funnel plots are not reliable) is misleading, as funnel plots are useful but should be interpreted alongside other tests like the **Egger test**.

## Advanced Surgical Talk

In meta-analysis, **publication bias** occurs when studies with significant results are more likely to be published, leading to skewed conclusions. To assess publication bias, researchers use **funnel plots** to visually check for symmetry and the **Egger test** to statistically assess bias. A **p-value** of less than **0.05** from the **Egger test** indicates potential bias, but borderline results (around 0.05) warrant caution in interpretation.

**Funnel plots** show whether the study results are symmetrically distributed around a midpoint line. Asymmetry in the plot may indicate publication bias, but this method is **subjective** and more reliable when used alongside statistical tests. Furthermore, both the funnel plot and Egger test are generally more reliable when there are at least **10 studies** in the analysis, as fewer studies may produce unreliable results.

In this scenario, with a **borderline Egger test p-value**, it's best to acknowledge the **possibility of bias** without making definitive conclusions [1][2].

Correct Answer: C) The results suggest possible publication bias, but the evidence is not definitive

**References**

1. Sterne JA, Egger M, Smith GD. Systematic reviews in health care: investigating and dealing with publication and other biases in meta-analysis. BMJ. 2001;323(7304):101-105.

2. Egger M, Davey Smith G, Schneider M, Minder C. Bias in meta-analysis detected by a simple, graphical test. BMJ. 1997;315(7109):629-634.

## Case 134: Types of Meta-Analyses

### Clinical Scenario

A research team is organizing a **meta-analysis** involving studies on a particular diagnostic test. They discuss the various types of meta-analyses, including **conventional**, **prognostic**, **diagnostic**, and **network meta-analyses**, and the conditions under which each type is appropriate.

### Question

Which type of meta-analysis involves combining **sensitivities** and **specificities** of diagnostic tests?

A) Conventional meta-analysis
B) Prognostic meta-analysis
C) Diagnostic meta-analysis
D) Network meta-analysis
E) Systematic review

### Explanation

A **diagnostic meta-analysis** is specifically designed to evaluate and combine the **diagnostic accuracy** of tests by pooling data on **sensitivities** and **specificities** across different studies. This type of meta-analysis is commonly used when evaluating the performance of diagnostic tests.

- **Option C is correct:** A **diagnostic meta-analysis** combines sensitivities and specificities to assess the overall diagnostic accuracy of a test.

- **Option A** (Conventional meta-analysis) typically combines effect sizes, not sensitivities and specificities.

- **Option B** (Prognostic meta-analysis) involves the combination of **hazard ratios** over time to evaluate **time-to-event outcomes**.

- **Option D** (Network meta-analysis) involves comparing interventions indirectly through a **common comparator** when direct comparisons are lacking.

- **Option E** (Systematic review) is a broader process that may include a meta-analysis, but it does not specifically involve combining diagnostic accuracy measures.

## Advanced Surgical Talk

Different types of **meta-analyses** are used depending on the nature of the data and the research question:

- A **conventional meta-analysis** typically combines **effect sizes** or outcomes from studies directly comparing interventions.

- A **prognostic meta-analysis** combines **time-based outcomes**, such as **hazard ratios**, to assess prognostic factors.

- A **diagnostic meta-analysis** focuses on pooling **sensitivity** and **specificity** data from diagnostic tests to assess their overall accuracy.

- A **network meta-analysis** allows comparisons of interventions that have not been directly compared in any single study by using a common comparator.

In this scenario, the researchers are focusing on the **diagnostic accuracy** of a test, making a **diagnostic meta-analysis** the most appropriate approach [1][2].

Correct Answer: C) Diagnostic meta-analysis

## References


1. Reitsma JB, Glas AS, Rutjes AW, et al. Bivariate analysis of sensitivity and specificity produces informative summary measures in diagnostic reviews. J Clin Epidemiol. 2005;58(10):982-990.

2. Riley RD, Ensor J, Snell KI, et al. Meta-analysis of diagnostic test studies using individual patient data and aggregate data. Stat Med. 2018;37(11):1705-1720.

## Clinical Scenario

You are tasked with producing a **meta-analysis** to evaluate the **survival benefits** of using **stents** versus **palliative chemotherapy** in patients with **metastatic cholangiocarcinoma**. During your literature search, you find:

- **6 studies** comparing **stents versus palliative chemotherapy**.

- **4 studies** comparing **stents versus radiotherapy**.

- No direct comparisons between **palliative chemotherapy** and **radiotherapy** are found.

## Question

Given the available studies, what is the most appropriate type of meta-analysis to perform?

A) Conventional meta-analysis
B) Prognostic meta-analysis
C) Diagnostic meta-analysis
D) Network meta-analysis
E) Systematic review without meta-analysis

## Explanation

A **network meta-analysis** is appropriate when there are **multiple treatment comparisons** that have not all been directly compared in head-to-head trials. In this case, you have studies comparing **stents vs palliative chemotherapy** and **stents vs radiotherapy**, but you do not have any studies directly comparing **palliative chemotherapy vs radiotherapy**.

A **network meta-analysis** allows you to make **indirect comparisons** between palliative chemotherapy and radiotherapy by using **stents** as the common comparator. This type of analysis is particularly useful when direct evidence is lacking but a connection can be made through a **shared comparator**.

- **Option D** is correct: A **network meta-analysis** is appropriate because it allows the indirect comparison of **palliative chemotherapy** and **radiotherapy** through the common comparator of **stents**.

- **Option A** (Conventional meta-analysis) would only compare two interventions directly and is not suitable for this scenario with three treatment arms.

- **Option B** (Prognostic meta-analysis) is used for studies involving time-to-event data, such as hazard ratios, but would not address indirect comparisons.

- **Option C** (Diagnostic meta-analysis) is focused on combining sensitivities and specificities of diagnostic tests, which is not relevant here.

- **Option E** (Systematic review without meta-analysis) might be used if no quantitative synthesis is possible, but in this case, a network meta-analysis is feasible.

**Advanced Surgical Talk**

A **network meta-analysis** is a powerful tool that allows for indirect comparisons between treatments that have not been directly compared in head-to-head studies. In this case, you have studies comparing **stents** with both **palliative chemotherapy** and **radiotherapy**, but no direct comparisons between **chemotherapy** and **radiotherapy**. The **network meta-analysis** approach uses the common comparator (stents) to assess the relative effectiveness of **chemotherapy vs radiotherapy**, even though no direct evidence is available.

This type of meta-analysis is particularly useful in situations like this, where multiple treatment options exist, but the literature does not fully cover all possible comparisons [1][2].

**Correct Answer: D) Network meta-analysis**

**References**

1. Mills EJ, Thorlund K, Ioannidis JP. Demystifying trial networks and network meta-analysis. BMJ. 2013;346.

2. Chaimani A, Caldwell DM, Li T, et al. Undertaking network meta-analyses. Cochrane Handbook for Systematic Reviews of Interventions. 2019.

## Clinical Scenario

A study is conducted to compare the **mean hospital stays** between two groups of patients. The data is **continuous** (hospital stay in days), and the distribution is assumed to be **normal** (parametric). The study involves **two independent samples** (patients in two different treatment groups).

## Question

What is the most appropriate statistical test to compare the **mean hospital stays** between these two groups?

A) Paired t-test
B) Mann-Whitney U test
C) Unpaired Student's t-test
D) Chi-square test
E) Wilcoxon signed-rank test

## Explanation

- The **mean hospital stay** is a **continuous variable**, and the assumption that it follows a **normal (parametric) distribution** implies the use of **parametric tests**.

- The data involves **two independent groups** (e.g., two different patient cohorts or treatment groups), making a **t-test** appropriate.

- Specifically, the **unpaired Student's t-test** is used when comparing the means of **two independent groups** for a continuous, normally distributed variable.

- **Option C is correct:** The **unpaired Student's t-test** is the most appropriate test for comparing the mean hospital stays between two independent groups.

- **Option A** (Paired t-test) is used for **paired** or **matched data**, such as when measurements are taken from the same individuals before and after an intervention.

- **Option B** (Mann-Whitney U test) is a **non-parametric** test, used when the data does not follow a normal distribution or when comparing **medians**.

- **Option D** (Chi-square test) is used for **categorical** data, not continuous data like hospital stays.

- **Option E** (Wilcoxon signed-rank test) is also a **non-parametric test**, used for **paired data**, not for comparing two independent samples.

## Advanced Surgical Talk

In clinical studies, choosing the correct statistical test is critical for proper data analysis. When dealing with **continuous data** (such as hospital stays) and assuming a **normal distribution**, parametric tests like the **unpaired Student's t-test** are used for comparing the means of two **independent groups**. If the data were not normally distributed, a **non-parametric test** like the **Mann-Whitney U test** would be more appropriate.

The **mean** is typically used for parametric data, while the **median** is used for non-parametric data. Since hospital stay is a **continuous variable**, understanding the distribution is key to selecting the correct statistical test [1][2].

Correct Answer: C) Unpaired Student's t-test

## References


1. Kim TK. T test as a parametric statistic. Korean J Anesthesiol. 2015;68(6):540-546.

2. Motulsky H. Common misconceptions about data analysis and statistics. Int J Clin Exp Pathol. 2007;4(1):123-127.


---

## Case 137: Statistical Test for Paired Data

### Clinical Scenario

A study is conducted to evaluate **pain scores** in a group of patients **before and after** an intervention. The pain scores are measured on a **continuous scale**, and the data is assumed to be **normally distributed** (parametric). The researchers want to compare the **mean pain scores** before and after the intervention within the **same group of patients**.

### Question

What is the most appropriate statistical test to compare the **mean pain scores** before and after the intervention in the same group of patients?

A) Paired Student's t-test
B) Unpaired Student's t-test
C) Mann-Whitney U test

D) Chi-square test

E) Wilcoxon signed-rank test

## Explanation

When comparing **before and after** data from the **same group of patients** (repeated measurements), the data is considered **paired**. Since the pain scores are **continuous** and **normally distributed** (parametric), the **paired Student's t-test** is the most appropriate statistical test to use.

- **Option A** is correct: The **paired Student's t-test** is used for comparing the means of **paired** or **related data** (e.g., measurements before and after an intervention in the same group).

- **Option B** (Unpaired Student's t-test) is used for comparing the means of **two independent groups**, not paired data.

- **Option C** (Mann-Whitney U test) is a **non-parametric test** used for comparing **independent groups** when the data is not normally distributed.

- **Option D** (Chi-square test) is used for **categorical** data, not continuous data like pain scores.

- **Option E** (Wilcoxon signed-rank test) is a **non-parametric test** for paired data, used when the assumption of normality is not met.

## Advanced Surgical Talk

The **paired Student's t-test** is the appropriate test when comparing **two related or paired samples**, such as measurements taken **before and after** an intervention in the same group of patients. In this scenario, both sets of pain scores (before and after the intervention) are from the same patients, and the data is assumed to be **parametric** (normally distributed).

If the data were **not normally distributed**, the **Wilcoxon signed-rank test** would be the appropriate non-parametric alternative. When dealing with continuous data and repeated measures, it's essential to account for the paired nature of the data to avoid incorrect conclusions [1][2].

Correct Answer: A) Paired Student's t-test

## References

1. Kim TK. T test as a parametric statistic. Korean J Anesthesiol. 2015;68(6):540-546.

2. Motulsky H. Common misconceptions about data analysis and statistics. Int J Clin Exp Pathol. 2007;4(1):123-127.

## Case 138: Fisher's Exact Test for Small Sample Sizes

### Clinical Scenario

A small study is conducted to compare the outcomes of two different treatments for a rare condition. The study involves only **20 patients**, and the outcomes are **categorical** (e.g., success or failure of the treatment). The research team wants to determine if there is a significant difference between the two treatments despite the small sample size.

### Question

What is the most appropriate statistical test to analyse the **categorical data** in this small sample size?

A) Chi-square test
B) Paired t-test
C) Fisher's exact test
D) Mann-Whitney U test
E) Unpaired t-test

### Explanation

The **Fisher's exact test** is used for analysing **categorical data**, especially when dealing with **small sample sizes**. It is often used when the **expected frequencies** in any cell of a contingency table are **less than 5**, making the **Chi-square test** unreliable. In this case, where the outcomes are **categorical** and the sample size is small, Fisher's exact test is the most appropriate statistical method.

- **Option C** is correct: **Fisher's exact test** is used for **categorical data** in small sample sizes.

- **Option A** (Chi-square test) is typically used for larger sample sizes and is less reliable when the sample size is small or expected frequencies are low.

- **Option B** (Paired t-test) is used for **continuous data** in paired samples, not for categorical data.

- **Option D** (Mann-Whitney U test) is a non-parametric test for **continuous data** between two independent groups.

- **Option E** (Unpaired t-test) is also used for **continuous data** between two independent groups.

## Advanced Surgical Talk

The **Fisher's exact test** is a powerful tool for analysing **categorical data** when the sample size is small. Unlike the **Chi-square test**, which assumes larger sample sizes and expected frequencies, Fisher's exact test can accurately determine whether there is a **significant association** between two categorical variables, even with very small numbers.

In studies with **small sample sizes** (often fewer than 30 subjects) or when the expected cell counts in a contingency table are less than 5, Fisher's exact test provides a more reliable result than the Chi-square test. It is widely used in **medical research** and other fields where sample sizes are often limited [1][2].

**Correct Answer: C) Fisher's exact test**

## References


1. Fisher RA. The logic of inductive inference. Journal of the Royal Statistical Society. 1935;98(1):39-82.

2. Kim HY. Statistical notes for clinical researchers: chi-squared test and Fisher's exact test. Restor Dent Endod. 2017;42(2):152-155.


---

## Case 139: Chi-Squared Test for Large Sample Sizes

### Clinical Scenario

A large study is conducted to compare the outcomes of two different treatments for a common condition. The study involves **200 patients**, and the outcomes are **categorical** (e.g., treatment success or failure). The research team wants to determine if there is a significant difference between the two treatments based on these outcomes.

### Question

What is the most appropriate statistical test to analyse the **categorical data** in this large sample size?

A) Fisher's exact test
B) Paired t-test
C) Chi-square test

D) Mann-Whitney U test

E) Unpaired t-test

## Explanation

The **Chi-square test** is the appropriate statistical test for analysing **categorical data** in **larger sample sizes**. It is commonly used to assess whether there is a significant association between two categorical variables (e.g., treatment success and failure between two groups). The test assumes that the **expected frequencies** in each cell of the contingency table are sufficiently large, typically greater than **5**.

- **Option C** is correct: The **Chi-square test** is used for analysing **categorical data** in **large sample sizes**.

- **Option A** (Fisher's exact test) is used for smaller sample sizes, especially when the expected frequencies in any cell are less than 5.

- **Option B** (Paired t-test) is for continuous data in paired samples, not for categorical data.

- **Option D** (Mann-Whitney U test) is a non-parametric test for continuous data between two independent groups.

- **Option E** (Unpaired t-test) is for continuous data between two independent groups.

## Advanced Surgical Talk

The **Chi-square test** is widely used in research for analysing relationships between **categorical variables** in large sample sizes. It tests whether the observed distribution of variables is significantly different from what is expected under the null hypothesis. For example, it can help determine whether two treatments lead to significantly different outcomes (e.g., success vs. failure) in a clinical study.

However, when sample sizes are small or when expected frequencies in a contingency table are less than **5**, the **Fisher's exact test** is more appropriate. This makes the **Chi-square test** better suited for **larger sample sizes**, as in the current scenario with 200 patients [1][2].

Correct Answer: C) Chi-square test

## References

1. McHugh ML. The Chi-square test of independence. Biochem Med (Zagreb). 2013;23(2):143-149.

2. Kim HY. Statistical notes for clinical researchers: chi-squared test and Fisher's exact test. Restor Dent Endod. 2017;42(2):152-155.

## Case 140: Non-Parametric Tests for Continuous Data

### Clinical Scenario

A study is conducted to assess **pain scores** in patients before and after a **knee replacement surgery**. The data on pain scores is **continuous**, but does not follow a normal distribution, making it **non-parametric**. The research team wants to use the appropriate statistical test to compare the pre- and post-surgery pain scores.

### Question

What is the most appropriate **non-parametric** statistical test to compare the **pain scores before and after** knee replacement surgery in the same group of patients?

A) Paired t-test
B) Mann-Whitney U test
C) Wilcoxon signed-rank test
D) Chi-square test
E) Fisher's exact test

### Explanation

The **Wilcoxon signed-rank test** is a **non-parametric test** used when comparing **paired or related data** (e.g., measurements before and after an intervention in the same group). It is used for **continuous data** that does not follow a normal distribution. In this case, the **pain scores before and after knee replacement** represent paired data, and since the data is non-parametric, the **Wilcoxon signed-rank test** is appropriate ( Table 9).

- **Option C is correct:** The **Wilcoxon signed-rank test** is used for comparing **paired non-parametric data**, such as pre- and post-surgery pain scores in the same patients.

- **Option A** (Paired t-test) is used for paired data but assumes a **normal distribution**, which is not the case here.

- **Option B** (Mann-Whitney U test) is a non-parametric test for **two independent samples**, not paired data.

- **Option D** (Chi-square test) is used for **categorical data**, not continuous data like pain scores.

- **Option E** (Fisher's exact test) is also used for categorical data, especially in small sample sizes.

**Advanced Surgical Talk**

When working with **continuous data** that does not follow a normal distribution, **non-parametric tests** are required. The **Wilcoxon signed-rank test** is the non-parametric equivalent of the **paired t-test** and is used to compare **two related or paired samples**. In contrast, the **Mann-Whitney U test** is used when comparing **two independent samples** of non-parametric continuous data.

In this scenario, since the **pain scores** are measured **before and after** surgery in the **same patients** (paired data), the **Wilcoxon signed-rank test** is the correct choice. This test ranks the differences between paired observations and tests whether the median of those differences is significantly different from zero [1][2].

**Correct Answer: C) Wilcoxon signed-rank test**

**References**


1. Fay MP, Proschan MA. Wilcoxon-Mann-Whitney or t-test? On assumptions for hypothesis tests and multiple interpretations of decision rules. Stat Surv. 2010;4:1-39.

2. Gibbons JD, Chakraborti S. Nonparametric Statistical Inference. 5th ed. CRC Press; 2010.


*Table 9: the appropriate statistical tests decisions based on the type of data*

| Category | Condition/Question | Action | Test |
| --- | --- | --- | --- |
| **Type of Data** | Continuous or Discrete (categorical) | Choose the appropriate analysis | Continuous or Chi-square tests for categorical data |
| **Type of Question** | Relationship or Differences | Depending on the data type | Regression, Correlation |

| | | | , ANOVA, t-tests |
| --- | --- | --- | --- |
| **Regressio n Analyses** | Do you have a true independent variable? | If yes, perform Regression Analyses | |
| **Correlatio n Analysis** | No independent variable | If no, perform Correlation Analysis | |
| **Parametri c vs Non- Parametri c** | Parametric assumptions satisfied? | Choose based on assumption s | Pearson's r for parametric, Spearman's Rank Correlation for non-parametric |
| **Difference s Between Groups** | What differences? | Tests for equal variances | Fmax test, Brown & Smythe's test, Bartlett's tests |
| **Two Groups** | Parametric assumptions satisfied? | Use t-tests | Student's unpaired t-test, Paired t-test (parametri c) |
| **Two Groups** (non-parametric) | Parametric assumptions not met | Use non-parametric tests | Mann-Whitney U or Wilcoxon Rank sums test |
| **More than Two Groups** | Parametric assumptions satisfied? | Use ANOVA or alternative test | ANOVA (parametri c) |

| More than Two Groups | Parametric assumptions not met | Use Kruskal-Wallis Test | Non-parametric test |
| --- | --- | --- | --- |
| **Post-hoc Analysis** | If significant result in ANOVA | Perform post-hoc analysis | Tukey's or Bonferroni's test (ANOVA), Dunn's Test (Kruskal-Wallis) |

## Standard Error vs. Standard Deviation

There is often **confusion** between **standard error (SE)** and **standard deviation (SD)**, but it is essential to understand that these are **two completely different statistics** used in different contexts and provide different types of information ( table 10).

**Standard Deviation (SD):**

- **Definition**: Standard deviation is a measure of the **spread** or **variability** within a **single dataset**. It tells us how much the individual data points in a sample or population deviate from the mean.

- **Context**: It is used to describe the **variability** of a sample or population. A larger SD means data points are more spread out, while a smaller SD means they are closer to the mean.

- **Example**: If you measure the height of 50 people and calculate the SD, you get a sense of how much individual heights vary from the average height.

**Standard Error (SE):**

- **Definition**: Standard error measures the **precision** of the sample **mean** (or other sample statistics) by indicating how much the sample mean is likely to vary from the true population mean.

- **Context**: It is used when making **inferences** about a population from a sample. SE decreases as sample size increases, indicating that a larger sample provides a more precise estimate of the population mean.

- **Formula**: SE = SD / √n (where "n" is the sample size).

- **Example**: If you take 50 random samples from a population and calculate the mean for each, the SE would tell you how much the sample means vary from the true population mean.

*Table 10: difference between standard error and standard deviation*

| Statistic | Definition | Context | Interpretation |
|---|---|---|---|
| **Standard Deviation** | Measures variability within a dataset | Describes the spread of data points in a sample | Indicates how spread out data points are |
| **Standard Error** | Measures precision of the sample mean | Used to estimate how close the sample mean is to the population mean | Decreases as sample size increases |

Understanding the difference between **standard error** and **standard deviation** is crucial in interpreting data analysis results correctly. **Standard deviation** provides information about the **spread** of data, while **standard error** tells us about the **reliability** of the sample mean as an estimate of the population mean.

---

## Case 41: Standard Error and Standard Deviation

### Clinical Scenario

A research team is conducting a study on the **effectiveness of a new drug** for lowering blood pressure. They collect data from **50 patients** and report the **mean blood pressure reduction** as **10 mmHg**, with a **standard deviation (SD)** of **2 mmHg**. One member of the team suggests that they should report the **standard error (SE)** instead of the **standard deviation** because it will make the results seem more precise. The team is now confused about which measure to report and when.

## Question

Which of the following statements is correct?

A) The standard error should be used to describe the variability within the sample.
B) The standard deviation should be used when making inferences about the population mean.
C) The standard deviation should be used to describe the spread of data in the sample.
D) The standard error is always larger than the standard deviation.
E) The standard deviation decreases as the sample size increases.

## Explanation

The **standard deviation (SD)** is used to describe the **variability** or **spread** of data points in a sample. It tells us how much the data points **deviate from the mean** within the sample itself. On the other hand, the **standard error (SE)** is used to describe the **precision** of the sample mean as an estimate of the **population mean** and decreases as the sample size increases.

- **Option C is correct:** The **standard deviation** should be used to describe the **spread** of data in the sample. It gives insight into how widely the data points are spread around the mean.

- **Option A is incorrect:** The **standard error** is not used to describe **variability**; it is used to estimate how close the sample mean is to the **population mean**.

- **Option B is incorrect:** When making inferences about the population mean, the **standard error** is used, not the **standard deviation**.

- **Option D is incorrect:** The **standard error** is always **smaller** than or equal to the **standard deviation**, because SE = SD / $\sqrt{n}$, where "n" is the sample size.

- **Option E is incorrect:** The **standard deviation** remains constant regardless of the sample size; it is the **standard error** that decreases as the sample size increases.

## Advanced Surgical Talk

Understanding the difference between **standard deviation (SD)** and **standard error (SE)** is crucial in data interpretation. The **standard deviation** measures the spread of individual data points, while the **standard error** provides insight into the precision of the sample mean as an estimate of the population mean.

- In clinical trials and other medical studies, **standard deviation** helps us understand the **variability** within the sample, showing how individual patients' outcomes deviate from the average.

- **Standard error**, on the other hand, decreases as the **sample size increases**, giving us more confidence that our sample mean is close to the true population mean.

In this case, reporting the **standard deviation** provides information about the **variability** of the blood pressure reduction within the sample, while the **standard error** would be used to show how precise the mean estimate is for the overall population [1][2].

**Correct Answer: C) The standard deviation should be used to describe the spread of data in the sample**

### References


1. Altman DG, Bland JM. Standard deviations and standard errors. BMJ. 2005;331(7521):903.

2. Nahm FS. Nonparametric statistical tests for the continuous data: the basic concept and the practical use. Korean J Anesthesiol. 2016;69(1):8-14.


## Case 142: One Sample Representing a Larger Population

### Clinical Scenario

A researcher is studying **hospital stay duration** in **50 patients** who have undergone **wide local excision** for **ductal carcinoma in situ (DCIS)**. The researcher calculates the **mean** hospital stay and the **standard deviation (SD)** for this sample. The researcher is aware that these **50 patients** are only a **representative sample** of the larger population of all patients with DCIS undergoing the same procedure worldwide. The goal is to use the data from this sample to **infer** information about the broader population of DCIS patients.

## Question

Which of the following statements best describes the researcher's situation?

A) The mean and standard deviation from the sample provide information only about the sample and cannot be used to make inferences about the population.
B) The mean from the sample is an exact estimate of the population mean.
C) The standard deviation from the sample is always larger than the population standard deviation.
D) The sample mean provides an estimate of the population mean, and the standard error quantifies how close the sample mean is likely to be to the population mean.
E) The standard error is used to describe the variability within the sample.

## Explanation

When a **sample** is used to represent a **larger population**, the **sample mean** is an **estimate** of the **population mean**, but it is not an exact value. The **standard error (SE)** helps to quantify how close the **sample mean** is likely to be to the **population mean**. The **standard deviation (SD)** describes the **variability** within the **sample** itself.

- **Option D** is correct: The **sample mean** provides an estimate of the **population mean**, and the **standard error** quantifies how close the sample mean is likely to be to the population mean.

- **Option A** is incorrect: The **sample statistics** (mean and SD) are used to **infer** information about the population, not just the sample.

- **Option B** is incorrect: The **sample mean** is an **estimate** of the population mean, not an exact measure.

- **Option C** is incorrect: The **sample standard deviation** is not necessarily larger than the **population standard deviation**; it depends on the sample and the population.

- **Option E** is incorrect: The **standard error** describes the precision of the **sample mean** in estimating the population mean, not the variability within the sample (which is described by the **standard deviation**).

## Advanced Surgical Talk

In clinical studies, it is crucial to understand that the data collected from a **sample** of patients (e.g., 50 patients) are used to make **inferences** about the **broader population**. The **sample mean** gives an estimate of the **population mean**, but due to the variability inherent in different samples, this estimate is not exact. The **standard error (SE)** helps to quantify how precise this estimate is by taking into account both the **standard deviation (SD)** and the **sample size**.

- **Larger sample sizes** will result in a smaller **standard error**, meaning the sample mean is likely to be closer to the population mean.

- **Smaller sample sizes** will result in a larger **standard error**, meaning there is more uncertainty about how close the sample mean is to the population mean.

Understanding the difference between **standard deviation** and **standard error** is important for interpreting study results and making accurate inferences about a larger population based on a sample.

Correct Answer: D) The sample mean provides an estimate of the population mean, and the standard error quantifies how close the sample mean is likely to be to the population mean.

---

## Case 143: Standard Error of the Mean

### Clinical Scenario

A study is conducted to evaluate the effect of a new medication on blood pressure. The sample consists of **196 patients**, and the **mean blood pressure reduction** is **10 mmHg** with a **standard deviation** of **2 mmHg**. The researchers want to calculate the **standard error (SE)** of the mean to understand the precision of their sample mean in estimating the population mean.

### Question

What is the **standard error (SE)** of the mean in this study?

A) 0.10
B) 0.12
C) 0.14

D) 0.20

E) 0.30

## Explanation

To calculate the **standard error of the mean (SE)**, use the following formula:

SE=Standard Deviation/Sample SizeSE = \frac{\text{Standard Deviation}}{\sqrt{\text{Sample Size}}}SE=Sample Size Standard Deviation

In this case:

- The **standard deviation (SD)** is **2 mmHg**.

- The **sample size (n)** is **196**.

1. First, calculate the **square root** of the sample size:

196=14\sqrt{196} = 14196=14

2. Next, divide the **standard deviation** by the square root of the sample size:

SE=2/14=0.14

## Final Answer:

The **standard error (SE)** of the mean is **0.14**.

## Advanced Surgical Talk

The **standard error** provides important information about how precisely the sample mean estimates the **population mean**. In this case, a **standard error of 0.14** indicates that the sample mean is a relatively precise estimate of the true population mean.

- A smaller **SE** suggests that the sample mean is likely to be **close to the population mean**, while a larger **SE** would suggest greater variability in the sample and a less precise estimate of the population mean.

Understanding the difference between **standard deviation** and **standard error** is crucial in clinical research. The **standard deviation** reflects the variability within the **sample**, while the **standard error** reflects the precision of the **sample mean** as an estimate of the **population mean**.

Correct Answer: C) 0.14

## Clinical Scenario

A regional cancer centre has gained a reputation for being highly effective in the treatment of a particular type of cancer. Over the last year, the centre has seen a large number of patients from surrounding regions, many of whom travelled long distances to seek care there. The team at the centre is concerned that their data may not be representative of the entire region. Additionally, they are conducting a study on a new screening test for early cancer detection, but they are aware of the risks of **lead time bias**.

## Question

Which of the following statements best describes the **biases** affecting the centre's data and screening study?

A) **Centripetal bias** occurs when patients tend to cluster around high-quality medical centres, which may not reflect the general population.
B) **Lead time bias** occurs when a new treatment makes patients live longer than expected.
C) **Centripetal bias** can be eliminated by increasing the sample size.
D) **Lead time bias** can be reduced by performing more frequent screenings.
E) **Centripetal bias** occurs when patients tend to cluster around local community hospitals.

## Explanation

- **Centripetal bias** occurs when patients gravitate towards **centres of excellence**, which can lead to data from that centre not being representative of the entire region or country. In this case, the large number of patients traveling to the **regional cancer centre** may cause the data to reflect a biased, potentially healthier or wealthier subset of the population.

- **Lead time bias** is a common issue in **screening studies**. It occurs when early detection of a disease (such as cancer) through screening makes it appear that patients live longer, even though the total survival time has not changed. This is because the disease was detected earlier, not because treatment has extended life.

- **Option A** is correct: **Centripetal bias** occurs when patients tend to cluster around high-quality medical centres, which may not reflect the general population.

- **Option B** is incorrect: **Lead time bias** refers to the earlier detection of disease through screening, not the efficacy of treatment.

- **Option C** is incorrect: Increasing the sample size does not eliminate **centripetal bias** because the sample still comes from a biased population (those who seek care at a centre of excellence).

- **Option D** is incorrect: More frequent screenings do not reduce **lead time bias**; they may actually exacerbate it.

- **Option E** is incorrect: **Centripetal bias** involves patients clustering around **centres of excellence**, not local hospitals.

**Advanced Surgical Talk**

In research, understanding and accounting for **biases** is crucial.

- **Centripetal bias** can skew the results of studies conducted at **centres of excellence** because the patient population may not reflect the overall population. This makes it difficult to generalize findings to the broader community. Patients seeking care at these centres may have better health awareness, resources, or access to care, which can affect outcomes.

- **Lead time bias** is especially problematic in **screening programs**. It makes a treatment or intervention appear more effective simply because the disease is detected earlier. In reality, **lead time bias** does not improve overall survival but only extends the period during which the patient is aware of the disease.

Researchers must carefully design studies to **account for these biases**, ensuring that their findings are valid and applicable to the larger population[1][2].

**Correct Answer: A) Centripetal bias occurs when patients tend to cluster around high-quality medical centres, which may not reflect the general population.**

## References

1.  McMahon PM, Gazelle GS, Louie AK. Biases in radiology and radiology research. AJR Am J Roentgenol. 2002;179(1):119-122.

2.  Welch HG, Schwartz LM, Woloshin S. Lead Time and Overdiagnosis in Cancer Screening. JAMA. 2000;285(8):897-902.

## Case 145: Lead Time Bias in Screening

### Clinical Scenario

A screening program for early detection of **prostate cancer** has been implemented in a community. The program is designed to detect the disease at an earlier stage than traditional diagnostic methods. After the program's introduction, patients diagnosed with prostate cancer appear to live longer than those diagnosed before the screening was available. However, researchers are concerned that this extended survival time might not reflect an actual improvement in outcomes, but rather an artifact of **lead time bias**.

### Question

Which of the following best describes **lead time bias**?

A) The screening process identifies patients who would otherwise have been missed.
B) The screening process leads to earlier detection, which falsely appears to increase survival time.
C) The treatment used after screening improves patient outcomes, leading to longer survival.
D) Lead time bias can be eliminated by using randomized control trials.
E) Lead time bias occurs when patients are diagnosed later in the disease course.

### Explanation

**Lead time bias** occurs when a **screening test** detects a disease earlier in its natural course, making it seem as though the patient lives longer after diagnosis. However, the **apparent increase in survival** is due to the fact that the disease was detected **earlier**, not because the treatment or outcomes were actually improved. This can make screening programs appear more effective than they are, even though the patient's overall prognosis may not have changed.

- **Option B** is correct: Lead time bias leads to the **earlier detection** of a disease, which falsely appears to increase survival time because the clock starts earlier.

- **Option A** is incorrect: While screening may identify patients who would otherwise be missed, this is not an example of lead time bias.

- **Option C** is incorrect: Lead time bias does not reflect improved outcomes from treatment; it reflects the earlier detection of the disease.

- **Option D** is incorrect: Randomized control trials can help evaluate the efficacy of screening programs, but they do not necessarily eliminate lead time bias.

- **Option E** is incorrect: Lead time bias refers to earlier, not later, diagnosis in the disease course.

## Advanced Surgical Talk

**Lead time bias** is an important consideration in evaluating the effectiveness of **screening programs**. A screening test may detect a disease earlier, giving the **illusion of increased survival**, even though the overall time from disease onset to death has not changed. This bias can overestimate the benefits of screening because patients may be living with the knowledge of their disease for a longer time, but without any real improvement in their prognosis.

To avoid the pitfalls of lead time bias, researchers need to focus on **overall mortality** and **quality of life outcomes** rather than just survival time after diagnosis. This ensures that the screening program is truly beneficial and not simply creating the appearance of longer survival due to earlier detection[1][2].

Correct Answer: B) The screening process leads to earlier detection, which falsely appears to increase survival time.

## References


1. Welch HG, Schwartz LM, Woloshin S. Lead Time and Overdiagnosis in Cancer Screening. JAMA. 2000;285(8):897-902.

2. Harris R, Sawaya GF, Moyer VA, Calonge N. Screening for prostate cancer: U.S. Preventive Services Task Force recommendation statement. Ann Intern Med. 2012;157(2):120-134.

## Clinical Scenario

A clinical trial is designed to test the effectiveness of a **weight loss program** that involves **exercise alone** as the intervention. The study recruits participants through advertisements in fitness magazines and online fitness forums. At the end of the trial, the researchers find that the weight loss results are significantly better than expected. However, they realize that the group of participants may not be representative of the general population of individuals who are trying to lose weight, as the participants seem to be highly motivated individuals with a pre-existing interest in fitness.

## Question

Which of the following best describes the bias affecting this study?

A) Selection bias occurs when the study group is not representative of the population that will be treated.
B) Lead time bias occurs when the disease is detected earlier in its course, falsely increasing survival.
C) Centripetal bias occurs when patients cluster around high-quality medical centres, skewing results.
D) Randomization can completely eliminate selection bias.
E) Attrition bias occurs when patients are lost to follow-up, impacting the study outcomes.

## Explanation

**Selection bias** occurs when the **study population** is not representative of the **general population** for which the treatment or intervention is intended. In this case, the participants are likely more **highly motivated** individuals with a strong interest in fitness, which may skew the results of the trial. As a result, the findings may not be generalizable to the broader population of people trying to lose weight, who may not be as motivated[1]

- **Option A is correct**: **Selection bias** occurs when the study group is not reflective of the population intended for the intervention. The patients in this study are likely more motivated, and the results may not apply to less motivated individuals.

- **Option B is incorrect**: **Lead time bias** occurs in screening studies and relates to the earlier detection of disease.

- **Option C** is incorrect: **Centripetal bias** refers to patients clustering around centres of excellence, which is unrelated to this study.

- **Option D** is incorrect: **Randomization** can reduce selection bias, but it cannot completely eliminate it if the study population is already skewed due to recruitment methods.

- **Option E** is incorrect: **Attrition bias** occurs when patients drop out of a study, which is not the issue here.

## Advanced Surgical Talk

**Selection bias** is a common issue in clinical research, especially when recruitment methods attract participants who may not be representative of the general population. In this case, individuals with a pre-existing interest in fitness were more likely to participate in the weight loss study, meaning the results may not apply to people who are less motivated or who face greater barriers to exercising.

- **Selection bias** can lead to **overestimation** or **underestimation** of the effectiveness of an intervention. In this scenario, the effectiveness of the weight loss program may appear better than it would be in a more diverse, less motivated population.

To minimize **selection bias**, researchers should use **randomized sampling methods** and ensure that their recruitment strategies reach a broad, representative sample of the target population[2].

**Correct Answer: A) Selection bias occurs when the study group is not representative of the population that will be treated.**

## References


1. Schulz KF, Grimes DA. Bias and causal associations in observational research. Lancet. 2002;359(9302):248-252.

2. Sedgwick P. Selection bias versus allocation bias. BMJ. 2013;346.

## Clinical Scenario

A researcher is conducting a study on the effects of a new drug for reducing **cholesterol levels**. The researcher strongly believes that the drug is effective and, during the analysis, gives more weight to the data points that show a significant reduction in cholesterol while downplaying or ignoring data that suggests no effect. As a result, the final conclusion supports the effectiveness of the drug, despite mixed evidence in the dataset.

## Question

Which of the following best describes the bias affecting this study?

A) Selection bias occurs when the study group is not representative of the population.
B) Confirmation bias occurs when the researcher interprets or selects information that supports their pre-existing beliefs.
C) Lead time bias occurs when a disease is detected earlier, falsely increasing survival time.
D) Attrition bias occurs when participants are lost to follow-up, impacting study results.
E) Centripetal bias occurs when patients cluster around high-quality medical centres, skewing results.

## Explanation

**Confirmation bias** occurs when researchers **selectively interpret** or **emphasize** data that supports their **preconceived beliefs** or **hypotheses**, while ignoring or downplaying data that contradicts them. In this case, the researcher wants the new drug to appear effective and therefore emphasizes the data that supports this view while ignoring data that does not [1].

- **Option B** is correct: **Confirmation bias** is when researchers use information to confirm or refute a hypothesis based on their preconceptions or desired outcomes.

- **Option A** is incorrect: **Selection bias** involves recruiting a non-representative sample, which is not the issue in this scenario.

- **Option C** is incorrect: **Lead time bias** is related to screening studies, where earlier detection can falsely appear to improve survival.

- **Option D** is incorrect: **Attrition bias** involves participants dropping out of a study, which is not applicable here.

- **Option E** is incorrect: **Centripetal bias** involves patients clustering around high-quality medical centres, not selectively interpreting data.

**Advanced Surgical Talk**

**Confirmation bias** is a major issue in scientific research and can lead to **misleading conclusions** if researchers unconsciously or consciously favor data that supports their pre-existing beliefs or hypotheses. This bias can occur at various stages of the research process, including:

- **Data collection**: Selectively gathering data that fits the desired outcome.

- **Data interpretation**: Giving more weight to findings that support the hypothesis.

- **Reporting**: Only publishing results that confirm the researcher's belief.

Researchers must remain objective and critically evaluate all data, regardless of whether it supports or refutes their initial hypothesis. Blind data analysis or having multiple investigators independently review the results can help reduce **confirmation bias** [2].

**Correct Answer: B) Confirmation bias occurs when the researcher interprets or selects information that supports their pre-existing beliefs.**

**References**


1. Nickerson RS. Confirmation bias: A ubiquitous phenomenon in many guises. Rev Gen Psychol. 1998;2(2):175-220.

2. Pohl RF. Cognitive illusions: A handbook on fallacies and biases in thinking, judgement and memory. Routledge; 2004.

## Clinical Scenario

A research study is designed to test the effectiveness of **gastric bypass surgery** on a group of patients. However, the study recruits patients with a **BMI of 20**, which is below the threshold typically used for such surgeries. Despite showing that gastric bypass surgery leads to weight loss in this group, the results are criticized because the patient population is not representative of those who would actually undergo the procedure in real life (patients with **severe obesity**).

## Question

Which of the following best describes the error in this study?

A) Type I error occurs when a true null hypothesis is rejected.

B) Type II error occurs when a false null hypothesis is accepted.

C) Type III error occurs when the research design or sample does not reflect actual practice.

D) Selection bias occurs when the study group is not representative of the population.

E) Attrition bias occurs when participants are lost to follow-up.

## Explanation

A **Type III error** occurs when there is a **model mis-specification**, meaning that the **research design, sample size,** or **demographic** does not reflect the reality of clinical practice. In this case, recruiting patients with a **BMI of 20** for **gastric bypass surgery** does not align with real-life clinical guidelines, which reserve the procedure for patients with **severe obesity** (typically BMI $\geq$ 40). Therefore, the study results are not applicable to the population that would typically undergo gastric bypass surgery.

- **Option C is correct:** A **Type III error** occurs when there is **model mis-specification** or a mismatch between the research design/sample and real-life practice.

- **Option A is incorrect:** A **Type I error** is rejecting a true null hypothesis, which is not relevant here.

- **Option B is incorrect:** A **Type II error** is accepting a false null hypothesis, which is not the issue here.

- **Option D** is incorrect: **Selection bias** refers to non-representative sampling, but in this case, it is more about choosing the wrong **type** of patients for the study.

- **Option E** is incorrect: **Attrition bias** refers to participants dropping out, which is not relevant in this scenario.

**Advanced Surgical Talk**

A **Type III error** occurs when the **study design** or **sample selection** is flawed, leading to results that are not applicable to the real-world population. In this scenario, performing gastric bypass surgery on patients with a **BMI of 20** is not reflective of **actual clinical guidelines**, which typically recommend the surgery for **patients with severe obesity** [1].

**Type III errors** can undermine the reliability of study results, as the conclusions drawn from such studies may not be generalizable to the intended patient population. Researchers need to ensure that their **sample population** and **study design** accurately reflect the **real-world context** in which the intervention would be applied[2].

Correct Answer: C) Type III error occurs when the research design or sample does not reflect actual practice.

**References**

1. Kim J, Smith JK. Type III errors in public health research: Avoiding the wrong problem in health care research and practice. JAMA. 2011;305(18):1886-1887.

2. Cleveland WS, Kleiner B, Tukey PA. Graphical methods for data presentation: Full-scale breaks, dot charts, and multibased logging. Am Stat. 1988;42(4):215-224.

## Case 149: Type II Error and Study Power

**Clinical Scenario**

A clinical trial is conducted to evaluate the effectiveness of a new **antibiotic** for treating **pneumonia**. The study fails to find a significant difference between the new antibiotic and the standard treatment. However, the researchers later realize that the study was **underpowered**, meaning the sample size was too small to detect a true difference if one existed. As a result, the trial incorrectly concludes that the new antibiotic is no better than the standard treatment.

## Question

Which of the following best describes the error in this study?

A) Type I error occurs when a true null hypothesis is rejected.
B) Type II error occurs when a false null hypothesis is accepted.
C) Type III error occurs when the research design or sample does not reflect actual practice.
D) Selection bias occurs when the study group is not representative of the population.
E) Centripetal bias occurs when patients cluster around high-quality medical centres.

## Explanation

A **Type II error** occurs when a study **fails to reject a false null hypothesis**. In this case, the study concluded that there was no difference between the new antibiotic and the standard treatment, but this conclusion may be incorrect due to **low statistical power**. **Power** is the probability that a study will detect an effect if there is one, and it depends on factors like **sample size** and **effect size**. An **underpowered** study is more likely to make a **Type II error**.

- **Option B** is correct: A **Type II error** occurs when the study inaccurately fails to reject the null hypothesis (i.e., accepts the null hypothesis when it is false).

- **Option A** is incorrect: A **Type I error** occurs when a true null hypothesis is incorrectly rejected, which is not the issue here.

- **Option C** is incorrect: A **Type III error** involves model mis-specification or a design that doesn't reflect actual practice.

- **Option D** is incorrect: **Selection bias** refers to a non-representative sample, which is not the issue in this study.

- **Option E** is incorrect: **Centripetal bias** involves patients clustering around centres of excellence, which is not relevant here.

## Advanced Surgical Talk

A **Type II error** occurs when a study **fails to detect a true effect** due to **insufficient statistical power**. This can happen when the **sample size** is too small or when the **effect size** is subtle. To minimize the risk of a **Type II error**, researchers need to ensure that the study is adequately **powered**, meaning the sample size is large enough to detect a meaningful difference if one exists.

- **Power** is typically set at **80% or higher**, meaning the study has at least an 80% chance of detecting an effect if it is present. Power can be increased by:
    - Increasing the **sample size**.
    - Increasing the **effect size** (e.g., choosing more sensitive outcome measures).
    - Reducing variability in the data (e.g., by improving measurement techniques).

In this case, the **underpowered** study was more likely to make a **Type II error**, leading to the incorrect conclusion that the new antibiotic was no more effective than the standard treatment [1][2].

**Correct Answer: B) Type II error occurs when a false null hypothesis is accepted.**

### References

1.  Button KS, Ioannidis JP, Mokrysz C, et al. Power failure: why small sample size undermines the reliability of neuroscience. Nat Rev Neurosci. 2013;14(5):365-376.

2.  Sedgwick P. Understanding statistical power. BMJ. 2015;350.

---

## Case 150: Appropriate Measure for Blood Loss

### Clinical Scenario

In a study evaluating blood loss during **elective surgery**, researchers collect data on the amount of blood lost by each patient. The data follows a **normal distribution**, meaning that most patients experience moderate blood loss, with fewer patients at the extremes (very low or very high blood loss). The research team is deciding which measure of central tendency—mean, median, or mode—would be the most appropriate to summarize the average blood loss in this study.

### Question

Which of the following is the most appropriate measure of central tendency to describe **average blood loss** in this scenario?

A) Mean
B) Median
C) Mode
D) Range
E) Interquartile Range (IQR)

## Explanation

When data follows a **normal distribution**, the **mean** is the most appropriate measure of central tendency. The **mean** takes into account all data points and provides the best estimate of the **average** for normally distributed data. In a normal distribution, the **mean**, **median**, and **mode** are all approximately equal, but the **mean** is the most informative measure for **parametric data**.

- **Option A** is correct: The **mean** is the most appropriate measure of central tendency for **normally distributed** data like blood loss.

- **Option B** is incorrect: The **median** is better for skewed data or non-normal distributions, but it is not needed when the data is normally distributed.

- **Option C** is incorrect: The **mode** represents the most frequent value and is less informative in a normal distribution.

- **Option D** is incorrect: The **range** describes the spread of the data, not the central tendency.

- **Option E** is incorrect: The **IQR** is a measure of spread, not central tendency, and is used for non-normally distributed data.

## Advanced Surgical Talk

In clinical research, the choice of the **central tendency** measure depends on the **distribution** of the data. For **normally distributed** data, such as blood loss in this study, the **mean** is the preferred choice because it incorporates all data points and provides an accurate representation of the central value.

If the data were **skewed** (e.g., if some patients had extremely high blood loss), the **median** would be more appropriate, as it is less affected by outliers. However, in this case of normally distributed data, the **mean** provides the most reliable estimate of **average blood loss**.

Correct Answer: A) Mean

# References


1. Altman DG, Bland JM. Statistics Notes: The normal distribution. BMJ. 1995;310(6975):298.

2. McHugh ML. The Chi-square test of independence. Biochem Med (Zagreb). 2013;23(2):143-149.

**Advanced Surgical Talks in FRCS: Mastering Techniques for Success**

The "Advanced Surgical Talks in FRCS: Mastering Techniques for Success" series is an essential collection for FRCS candidates, meticulously crafted to align with the current FRCS examination format. Each book in this comprehensive series delves into a specific surgical discipline, providing in-depth knowledge, updated references, and the latest guidelines. The series includes:

- **Breast Surgery**
- **Endocrine Surgery**
- **General Surgery**
- **Traumatology**
- **Gastrointestinal Surgery**
- **Colorectal Surgery**
- **Hepatobiliary Surgery**
- **Emergency Surgery**
- **Critical Care**
- **Transplant Surgery**
- **Vascular Surgery**

Authored by experts in the field, these volumes are designed to equip candidates with the crucial insights and advanced techniques needed to excel in their examinations and professional practice. With a focus on single best answer MCQs, this series offers a thorough understanding of surgical principles and practices, ensuring that readers are well-prepared for success. Perfect for both study and reference, "Advanced Surgical Talks in FRCS" is a must-have resource for aspiring surgeons committed to achieving excellence in their field.

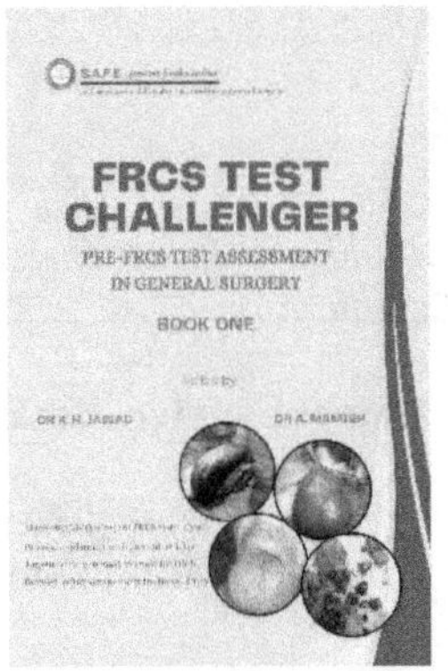

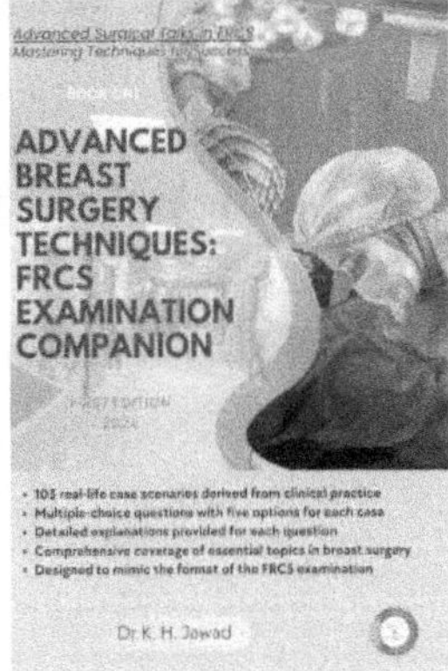

<u>**Advanced Breast Surgery Techniques: FRCS Examination Companion**</u>

Preparing for the FRCS (Fellowship of the Royal Colleges of Surgeons) examination  requires a comprehensive and strategic approach. Here are some general tips to help you prepare effectively:

**1.** Understand the Exam Structure:

- Familiarize yourself with the format of the exam, including the different components (written, clinical, viva).

- Know the specific requirements for each section.

**2.** Create a Study Schedule:

- Develop a realistic and structured study schedule. Allocate time for each subject or topic, ensuring comprehensive coverage.

- Include breaks to avoid burnout.

**3.** Identify Weaknesses and Strengths:

- Assess your strengths and weaknesses in each subject area.

- Allocate more time to areas where you need improvement.

**4.** Use Recommended Resources:

- Utilize official FRCS syllabus and recommended textbooks.

- Stay updated with the latest guidelines and research in your field.

**5.** Practice Past Papers:

- Work through past examination papers to familiarize yourself with the format and question types.

- Practice time management to ensure you can answer all questions within the allocated time.

**6.** Clinical Skills Practice:

- For clinical and viva components, practice your clinical skills regularly.

- Seek opportunities for hands-on experience and exposure to a variety of cases.

**7.** Stay Informed:

- Keep yourself updated with the latest developments and research in your field.

- Attend relevant conferences, workshops, and seminars.

**8.** Join Study Groups:

- Form or join study groups to discuss and review topics with peers.

- Engage in discussions to enhance your understanding of different

perspectives.

**9.** Seek Feedback:

- Request feedback from mentors, colleagues, or supervisors on your performance during mock exams or practice sessions.

**10.**Maintain a Healthy Lifestyle:

- Ensure you get enough sleep, exercise, and maintain a balanced diet to support your overall well-being.

- Manage stress through relaxation techniques.

**11.**Simulate Exam Conditions:

- Practice under exam conditions to get accustomed to the pressure and time constraints.

## List of Abbreviations:

- AAA (Abdominal Aortic Aneurysm)
- ACS (Abdominal Compartment Syndrome)
- AHS (Abdominal Hernia Surgery)
- AJCC (American Joint Committee on Cancer)
- AKI (Acute Kidney Injury)
- ASA (American Society of Anaesthesiologists)
- BCC (Basal Cell Carcinoma)
- BMI (Body Mass Index)
- CBD (Common Bile Duct)
- CDAD (Clostridium Difficile-Associated Diarrhoea)
- CI (Confidence Interval)
- CMV (Cytomegalovirus)
- CNS (Central Nervous System)
- COPD (Chronic Obstructive Pulmonary Disease)
- CPET (Cardiopulmonary Exercise Testing)
- CRP (C-Reactive Protein)
- CT (Computed Tomography)
- CVP (Central Venous Pressure)
- DIC (Disseminated Intravascular Coagulation)
- DVT (Deep Vein Thrombosis)
- EBV (Epstein-Barr Virus)
- EHS (European Hernia Society)

- FN (False Negative)

- FP (False Positive)

- FRCS (Fellowship of the Royal Colleges of Surgeons)

- GCS (Glasgow Coma Scale)

- GI (Gastrointestinal)

- GMC (General Medical Council)

- HIT (Heparin-Induced Thrombocytopenia)

- ICU (Intensive Care Unit)

- IQR (Interquartile Range)

- LAST (Local Anaesthetic Systemic Toxicity)

- LMWH (Low-Molecular-Weight Heparin)

- MALT (Mucosa-Associated Lymphoid Tissue)

- MAP (Mean Arterial Pressure)

- MDT (Multidisciplinary Team)

- MI (Myocardial Infarction)

- MRI (Magnetic Resonance Imaging)

- NNT (Number Needed to Treat)

- NPV (Negative Predictive Value)

- OR (Odds Ratio)

- PCA (Patient-Controlled Analgesia)

- PCR (Polymerase Chain Reaction)

- PPV (Positive Predictive Value)

- ROC (Receiver Operating Characteristic)

- RSI (Rapid Sequence Induction)

- SCC (Squamous Cell Carcinoma)

- SD (Standard Deviation)

- SE (Standard Error)

- SSI (Surgical Site Infection)

- TAP (Transversus Abdominis Plane)

- TXA (Tranexamic Acid)

- USS (Ultrasound Scan)

- UV (Ultraviolet)

- VTE (Venous Thromboembolism)

- WHO (World Health Organization)

# Index